Consumer-Run Mental Health

Louis D. Brown

Consumer-Run Mental Health

Framework for Recovery

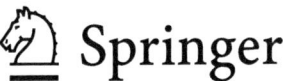 Springer

Louis D. Brown, Ph.D.
University of Texas School of Public Health
El Paso, TX, USA
louis.d.brown@uth.tmc.edu

ISBN 978-1-4614-0699-0   e-ISBN 978-1-4614-0700-3
DOI 10.1007/978-1-4614-0700-3
Springer New York Dordrecht Heidelberg London

Library of Congress Control Number: 2011937236

© Springer Science+Business Media, LLC 2012
All rights reserved. This work may not be translated or copied in whole or in part without the written permission of the publisher (Springer Science+Business Media, LLC, 233 Spring Street, New York, NY 10013, USA), except for brief excerpts in connection with reviews or scholarly analysis. Use in connection with any form of information storage and retrieval, electronic adaptation, computer software, or by similar or dissimilar methodology now known or hereafter developed is forbidden.
The use in this publication of trade names, trademarks, service marks, and similar terms, even if they are not identified as such, is not to be taken as an expression of opinion as to whether or not they are subject to proprietary rights.

Printed on acid-free paper

Springer is part of Springer Science+Business Media (www.springer.com)

This book is dedicated to the P.S. Club and all of its members for having the courage to share their story with the world.

Preface

This book seeks to develop and explore an integrated theoretical framework called the role framework, which explains how involvement in mental health consumer-run organizations (CROs) can promote recovery. Given the book's emphasis on theory, it will primarily appeal to researchers who study consumer-run organizations and self-help. However, parts of this book can be useful to several other audiences. Students studying psychiatric diagnoses can use the accessible journalistic life history narratives and documentary photography to gain insight into the lived experience of developing and recovering from mental health problems. Rather than categorizing people with descriptions of symptoms, the narratives provide an insider's perspective on the development of mental health problems and the process of recovery. Mental health consumers may find the narratives inspiring because some of the featured consumers have made great progress towards recovery and also useful because the narratives share problem-solving strategies that others have used successfully.

This book may also appeal to several audiences outside of those directly interested in CROs, mental health problems, and recovery. Social psychologists may be interested in my novel application of identity theory. Researchers interested in theory development may be interested in my use of focused questions to develop the role framework. Qualitative researchers may be interested in the use of journalistic narratives as a research methodology because narratives can help to bridge the gap between research and practice by providing research findings that appeal to a broader audience.

Before readers judge the accuracy, validity, and usefulness of this work, it is helpful to consider several issues. First, I have an unique perspective that has substantially influenced the contents of this book, just as all writers' perspectives influence their work. My hope is that readers judge my work on its believability after critical inspection rather than the pureness of its objectivity. My subjective perspective has influenced this research in innumerable ways. Although I do not have insight into all of my subjective influences, I explain some important influences in the following paragraphs.

First, when I began writing this book, I was convinced mental health consumer-run organizations (CROs) were a good idea. The intention of this work is not to prove that CROs are effective. Instead the studies presented in this book were intended to generate a robust theoretical for understanding how CROs can help to promote recovery. The efficacy and cost effectiveness of CROs remain important research questions. As such, I review the relevant research in this book, which makes it clear CROs can be beneficial. This book focuses on understanding how CROs can be beneficial.

Much of the research presented in this book is grounded in the insider's perspective, which has an important impact on the results. The people who go to CROs believe they are helpful; otherwise they would not attend. Further, members create and maintain an organization out of their own free will, making them unlikely to criticize the organization's existence. Thus, consideration of the insider perspective provides a favorable understanding of CROs. This book seeks to develop a generalizable theoretical framework that remains congruent with an insider's perspective, explaining both the nature of the CRO participation experience and how it changes the people who experience it. However, it is important to note that I do not intend to glaze over the problematic realities of CROs. Like any organization, CROs face formidable challenges and this work addresses important problems and limitations of CROs.

A second issue to consider before critically digesting this work is that I do not believe our social world is grounded in objective reality in the same way as physical objects. Relationships between people are abstractions. They are fundamental to our existence and yet each mind perceives each relationship differently. Ideally people reach a shared understanding of their relationship, but that understanding changes over time and is never entirely synchronized. Thus, there is no way to objectively study the social world behind our social behavior. Analysis will always be the product of rationality and logic grounded in subjective experience and perspective. Although this work is not objective, I hope it remains useful. My reasoning and logic in the development of a theoretical framework is as much art as science. Nevertheless, I hope readers find the work to be based on sound evidence and logic rather than vacuous rationalization.

El Paso, TX   Louis D. Brown

Acknowledgments

Support for research presented in this book comes from the Kansas Department of Social and Rehabilitation Services, Division of Mental Health and NIMH (grant number 5T32MH018834-18). I would like to thank Matt Shepherd for his help with data collection and Greg Meissen, Lou Medvene, Sharon Iorio, Deac Dorr, and Darcee Datteri for their feedback on earlier versions of this work. I am grateful for the transcription support of Dorian Soto and Ellen Hudson. Many thanks also go to Amanda Applegate, whose timely editorial support helped to improve the clarity and readability of the book.

This book serves as a culmination and integration of numerous studies. Many of the studies have been published as journal articles or book chapters in collaboration with several supporting authors. I would like to thank Matt Shepherd, Scott Wituk, Greg Meissen, Ed Merkle, and Alicia Lucksted for their help in conceptualizing, executing, and writing up these previously published journal articles and book chapters.

Following is a list of publications from which this book draws excerpts.

Brown, L.D. & Wituk, S.A. (2010). Introduction to mental health self-help. In L.D. Brown & S.A. Wituk (Eds.), *Mental health self-help: Consumer and family initiatives* (pp. 1–18). New York: Springer. Excerpts used with kind permission from Springer Science + Business Media: Mental Health self-help: Consumer and family initiatives, Introduction to mental health self-help, 2010, pp. 1–18, Louis Brown and Scott Wituk, ©Springer Science + Business Media, LLC 2010.

Brown, L.D. & Lucksted, A. (2010). Theoretical foundations of mental health self-help. In L.D. Brown & S.A. Wituk (Eds.), *Mental health self-help: Consumer and family initiatives* (pp. 19–38). New York: Springer. Excerpts used with kind permission from Springer Science + Business Media: Mental health self-help: Consumer and family initiatives, Theoretical foundations of mental health self-help, 2010, pp. 19–38, Louis Brown and Alicia Lucksted, ©Springer Science+Business Media, LLC 2010.

Brown, L.D., Wituk, S.A., & Meissen, G. (2010). Consumer-run drop-in centers: Current state and future directions. In L.D. Brown & S.A. Wituk (Eds.), *Mental health self-help: Consumer and family initiatives* (pp. 155–168). New York: Springer.

Excerpts used with kind permission from Springer Science+Business Media: Mental health self-help: Consumer and family initiatives, Consumer-run drop-in centers: Current state and future directions, 2010, pp. 155–168, Louis Brown, Scott Wituk, and Greg Meissen, ©Springer Science+Business Media, LLC 2010.

Brown, L.D. (2009). How people can benefit from mental health consumer-run organizations. *American Journal of Community Psychology, 43,* 177–188. Excerpts used with kind permission from Springer Science+Business Media: American Journal of Community Psychology, How people can benefit from mental health consumer-run organizations, Volume 43, 2009, 177–188, Louis Brown, ©Springer Science+Business Media, LLC 2009.

Brown, L.D. (2009). Making it sane: Using life history narratives to explore theory in a mental health consumer-run organization. *Qualitative Health Research, 19,* 243–257. The final, definitive version of this paper has been published in Qualitative Health Research, Volume 19 Number 2, February 2009 by Sage Publications, All rights reserved. ©http://qhr.sagepub.com/ hosted at http://online.sagepub.com

Brown, L.D., Shepherd, M.D., Merkle, E.C., Wituk, S.A., & Meissen, G. (2008). Understanding how participation in a consumer-run organization relates to recovery. *American Journal of Community Psychology, 42,* 167–178. Excerpts used with kind permission from Springer Science+Business Media: American Journal of Community Psychology, Understanding how participation in a consumer-run organization relates to recovery, Volume 42, 2008, 167–178, Louis Brown, Matt Shepherd, Edgar Merkle, Scott Wituk, and Greg Meissen, ©Springer Science+Business Media, LLC 2008.

Brown, L.D., Shepherd, M.D., Wituk, S.A., & Meissen, G. (2008). Introduction to the special issue on mental health self-help. *American Journal of Community Psychology, 42,* 105–109. Excerpts used with kind permission from Springer Science+Business Media: American Journal of Community Psychology, Introduction to the special issue on mental health self-help, Volume 42, 2008, 105–109, Louis Brown, Matt Shepherd, Scott Wituk, and Greg Meissen, ©Springer Science+Business Media, LLC 2008.

Brown, L.D., Shepherd, M.D., Wituk, S.A., & Meissen, G. (2007a). How settings change people: Applying behavior setting theory to consumer-run organizations. *Journal of Community Psychology, 35,* 399–416. The final, definitive version of this paper has been published in the Journal of Community Psychology, Volume 35 Number 3, April 2007 by Wiley InterScience (http://www.interscience.wiley.com), ©2007 Wiley Periodicals, Inc.

Brown, L.D., Shepherd, M.D., Wituk, S.A., & Meissen, G. (2007b). Goal achievement and the accountability of consumer-run organizations. *Journal of Behavioral Health Services and Research, 34,* 73–82. Excerpts used with kind permission from Springer Science+Business Media: Journal of Behavioral Health Services and Research, Volume 34, 2007, 73–82, Louis Brown, Matt Shepherd, Scott Wituk, and Greg Meissen, ©Springer Science+Business Media, LLC 2007.

Contents

1 Introduction 1
    Defining Qualities of CROs 3
    History of CROs and Mental Health Care 4
    Research on the Effectiveness of CROs 6
    Organizational Dynamics 7
        Organizational Structure 8
        Organizational Capacity Needs and Technical Assistance 10
        Factors Influencing the Use of CROs 10
        Funding Support and Avoiding Cooptation 11
        Interorganizational Relations 12
        Shared Leadership 13
    Overview of the Book 13

2 Using Existing Theory to Build a Conceptual Framework of Consumer-Run Organizations 15
    Part 1: Conceptualization of CRO Outcomes 17
        1A. Recovery 17
        1B. Community Integration 18
        1C. Sense of Community/Psychological Integration 19
    Part 2: Setting Characteristic Theories 20
        2A. Behavior-Setting Theory 20
        2B. Empowerment Theory 22
    Part 3: Interpersonal Processes Within CROs 23
        3A. The Helper-Therapy Principle 23
        3B. Experiential Knowledge 23
        3C. Social Comparison Theory 24
        3D. Social Support Theories 25
    Part 4: Roles and Identity Theory 26
    Part 5: The Preliminary Framework 29
        Component One: Person–Environment Interaction 30
        Component Two: Role and Relationship Development 31

Component Three: Build Role Skills	32
Component Four: Identity Transformation	32
Relating the Preliminary Explanatory Framework to Other Theoretical Perspectives	33
Improving the Preliminary Theoretical Framework	34

3 Refining the Preliminary Framework to Create the Role Framework 35

Focused Questions Methodology	36
Study Setting	36
Data Collection Procedure	37
Study Sample	37
Data Analysis	38
Categories and Causes of Personal Change	39
Integrating Categories to Create the Role Framework	41
Person–Environment Interaction	41
Role and Relationship Development	42
Resource Exchange	43
Self-Appraisal	44
Building Role Skills	44
Identity Transformation	45
Discussion	45
Connecting Framework Revisions to the Existing Literature	46
Limitations and Future Research	47
Conclusions	47

4 Constructing Journalistic Life History Narratives to Explore the Role Framework 49

Conceptual and Epistemological Foundations of Narrative	50
Narratives as a Research Methodology	51
Integrating Journalism and Ethnographic Research	52
Visual Storytelling	53
Study Setting: The P.S. Club	53
Study Sample	54
Participant Observation	55
Minimally Structured Interviews	57
Life History Construction	58
Analysis of Narratives	60
Sharing Narratives	61
Conclusion	61

5 Life History Narratives from the P.S. Club 63

Life Inside Wellington's Mental Health System	63
Facing Serious Mental Health Problems, Running a Nonprofit	68
Mary's Story	82
Nick's Story	87
Carl's Story	94

Contents   xiii

    Joe's Story 98
    Kevin's Story 102
    Laura's Story 109
    Sue's Story 112

**6 Using Narratives to Understand How People Benefit
from CROs** 119
    Theoretical Analysis of Mary 119
        Component One: Person–Environment Interaction 119
        Component Two: Role and Relationship Development 120
        Component Three: Resource Exchange 120
        Component Four: Self-Appraisal 120
        Component Five: Building Role Skills 121
        Component Six: Identity Transformation 121
    Theoretical Analysis of Nick 121
        Component One: Person–Environment Interaction 121
        Component Two: Role and Relationship Development 121
        Component Three: Resource Exchange 122
        Component Four: Self-Appraisal 122
        Component Five: Building Role Skills 122
        Component Six: Identity Transformation 123
    Theoretical Analysis of Carl 123
        Component One: Person–Environment Interaction 123
        Component Two: Role and Relationship Development 123
        Component Three: Resource Exchange 124
        Component Four: Self-Appraisal 124
        Component Five: Building Role Skills 124
        Component Six: Identity Transformation 124
    Theoretical Analysis of Joe 125
        Component One: Person–Environment Interaction 125
        Component Two: Role and Relationship Development 125
        Component Three: Resource Exchange 125
        Component Four: Self-Appraisal 126
        Component Five: Building Role Skills 126
        Component Six: Identity Transformation 126
    Theoretical Analysis of Kevin 126
        Component One: Person–Environment Interaction 126
        Component Two: Role and Relationship Development 127
        Component Three: Resource Exchange 127
        Component Four: Self-Appraisal 127
        Component Five: Building Role Skills 127
        Component Six: Identity Transformation 128
    Theoretical Analysis of Laura 128
        Component One: Person–Environment Interaction 128
        Component Two: Role and Relationship Development 128
        Component Three: Resource Exchange 128

	Component Four: Self-Appraisal	129
	Components Five and Six: Building Role Skills and Identity Transformation	129
	Theoretical Analysis of Sue	129
	Component One: Person–Environment Interaction	129
	Component Two: Role and Relationship Development	130
	Component Three: Resource Exchange	130
	Component Four: Self-Appraisal	130
	Component Five: Building Role Skills	131
	Component Six: Identity Transformation	131
	Summary Cross-Case Analysis of Life History Narratives	132
	Component One: Person–Environment Interaction	132
	Component Two: Role and Relationship Development	132
	Component Three: Resource Exchange	133
	Component Four: Self-Appraisal	133
	Component Five: Building Role Skills	133
	Component Six: Identity Transformation	134
	Limitations and Future Research	134
	Conclusion	134
7	**How Organizations Influence Role Development**	137
	Organizational Size	138
	Leadership Involvement	138
	Recovery	139
	Study Hypotheses	140
	Method	140
	CRO Quarterly Reports	141
	Organizational Activity Survey	141
	Organizational Health Survey	141
	Results	142
	Discussion	145
	How Organizational Size Influences Leadership Role Development	145
	How Leadership Role Development Influences Recovery	146
	Shortcomings of Behavior Setting Theory	147
	Integrating the Role Framework and Behavior Setting Theory	148
	How the Role Framework Can Address Several Criticisms of Behavior Setting Theory	148
	Limitations and Future Research	149
	Conclusions	150
8	**Role Development and Recovery**	151
	Role Development and Recovery	152
	Relating Friendship and Leadership Roles	153
	Study Overview and Hypotheses	153

	Method	154
	Measures	154
	Statistical Methods	155
	Results	156
	Hypothesis 1	158
	Hypothesis 2	158
	The Social Networks of CRO Members	158
	Interpretation of Results	159
	Promoting an Empowering Environment	160
	Volunteer Opportunities	160
	Organizational Decision Making	160
	Planning and Organizing Activities	161
	Formal Leadership Positions	161
	Promoting a Socially Supportive Environment	161
	Recognize Member Accomplishments	162
	Organize a Variety of Interesting Activities	162
	Prevent and Resolve Conflict with a Code of Conduct	162
	Develop Self-Help Groups and/or Peer Counselors	163
	Comparing Friendship and Leadership Roles	164
	Limitations and Future Research	164
	Conclusions	166
9	**Conclusion**	167
	General Insights into the Recovery Process	167
	Summary Implications for Practice	169
	Developing Challenging New Roles	169
	Readiness for Challenging New Roles	170
	Recreation and Social Support	170
	Conflict	171
	Promoting the Development of Leadership and Friendship Roles	171
	Organizational Size	172
	Strengths and Weaknesses of the Methods	172
	Future Research Directions	174
	Closing Remarks	178
Appendix A		181
Appendix B		189
Appendix C		195
Appendix D		201
References		203
Index		215

Chapter 1
Introduction

Abstract Consumers of traditional mental health services receive help in dependency roles that have low status and power. In the public mental health system, these dependency roles can lead to learned helplessness, where consumers earn the care they receive by continually failing to care for themselves. Mental health consumer-run organizations (CROs) help to combat the problem of learned helplessness by providing consumers opportunities to help themselves and help others through their involvement in a consumer-controlled nonprofit. This book seeks to develop an improved understanding of how people benefit from CROs. The introductory chapter reviews the history of CROs, moving from their grassroots self-help group beginnings to the myriad of services CROs have started providing. The chapter reviews evidence on effectiveness of CROs that operate drop-in centers, which are the focus of this book. Several important organizational dynamics are considered, including organizational structure, organizational capacity needs, funding support, interorganizational relations, and shared leadership. Finally, the chapter concludes by providing an overview of the remaining book chapters.

In her ethnography, *Making it Crazy*, Estroff (1985) stated the contradictions of treatment in the traditional mental health system. In order to get well, you need help. In order to get help, you must prove your incompetence. Once proven, you will receive care, inadvertently but persistently reminding you of your incompetence. During care, you will be expected to try to take care of yourself. As long as you periodically try and fail to take care of yourself, you will continue to prove your incompetence and qualify for the care you are receiving. If you prove to be competent, you will stop qualifying for care. Such are the reciprocal rights and obligations in the role of a mental health patient.

Mental health consumer-run organizations (CROs) stand as an alternative to this paradox. Instead of occupying dependency or sick roles, people support each other as equals, both working and playing together. Rather than pity for the helpless, there is empathy for the struggle. The tedium of sheltered workshops is replaced with the personally meaningful task of maintaining an organization that is yours. With time, individuals start *making it sane* in life as people who can help themselves and help others in a similar situation.

Building on this foundational idea of creating strengths-based roles for people with mental health problems rather than dependency roles, this book seeks to develop a more refined understanding of how people benefit from CROs. Although the nature of CROs is varied, these organizations are defined first and foremost as nonprofit operated and controlled by people with mental health problems. As discussed in detail later in this introductory chapter, the emphasis of CROs on mutual support is similar to that of a self-help group, but they generally maintain more organizational structure than self-help groups.

CROs are an important part of the mental health system because they are a low cost strategy for promoting the well-being of mental health consumers with a strong evidence base supporting their effectiveness (Nelson, Ochocka, Janzen, & Trainor, 2006; Segal, Silverman, & Temkin, 2010; Teague, Johnsen, Rogers, & Schell, 2005). Despite receiving little funding support, over 4,000 CROs operate in the United States, of which 1,400 maintain drop-in centers (Goldstrom et al., 2006). Although CROs are popular, cost-efficient, and have a strong evidence base, many questions about the nature of CRO participation and its consequences remain. Insights from this book can inform the development of effective CROs that successfully engage participants in wellness-enhancing roles. In-depth analysis of how CROs fit into the larger mental health system also provides insight into the development of effective policies and support systems that help to ensure that publically funded CROs are successful.

To enhance understanding of how people benefit from CROs, this book aims to develop and explore a quantitatively testable theoretical framework that can connect the ideas of existing theoretical explanations in the literature, account for a broad array of CRO participation outcomes, and remain grounded in lived experience. I initially develop a framework through consideration of existing theory and the analysis of responses to focused questions about how CRO participation is beneficial. The result is the role framework, which provides a structural and psychological explanation of how people benefit from CROs and can more generally provide insight into the causes and consequences of role and relationship development in community settings.

To gain further insight into the nature of CRO participation and the utility of the role framework, I used ethnographic and journalistic data collection techniques. From these data, I created journalistic life history narratives of CRO participants, which combine with documentary photography to create an ethnographic look at life inside a nonprofit operated by people with severe mental health problems. The colorful narratives and images illustrate how the troubled lives of participants improve through their involvement in the organization. Analyzing life history narratives using the role framework provides new insights into both the lives of informants and the theoretical model. The book also presents results from quantitative studies examining different aspects of the role framework. The first set of analyses uses multilevel regression models to understand how organizational characteristics influence the development of roles.

The second set of analyses uses structural equation models to examine the relation between involvement in different organizational roles and recovery.

A more complete understanding of CROs can be useful to a variety of audiences including CRO leaders, potential members, mental health professionals, policy makers, and researchers. CRO leaders can use this information to better understand how their organization needs to be structured in order to be beneficial to members. Potential members can use this information to evaluate whether CRO participation would be beneficial to them. Mental health professionals can use an improved understanding of CROs to better assess which of their clients may benefit from a referral. Professionals can also use the information to better support and collaborate with CROs. Policy makers who understand how and why CROs are beneficial can make better decisions about how to support CROs. Finally, researchers can use the improved theoretical understanding to design evaluations and measures that are consistent with the theorized processes and outcomes of CRO participation.

The remaining sections of this chapter examine the defining qualities of CROs, review their historical development, and explicate the paradigm shift in the public mental health system towards consumer control, autonomy, mutual support, and recovery. This chapter also reviews research on the effectiveness of CROs and discusses organizational challenges and strategies for success. Finally, this introductory chapter provides an overview of the book as a whole and each chapter to come.

Defining Qualities of CROs

Since deinstitutionalization began, people with mental health problems and their families have been organizing a wide range of initiatives, including self-help groups, coalitions, nonprofit organizations, and businesses (Kimura, Mukaiyachi, & Ito, 2002; McLean, 2000; Mowbray, Chamberlin, Jennings, & Reed, 1988). These collaborative efforts directed by mental health consumers and their caregivers are called mental health self-help (Brown & Wituk, 2010). Although this book focuses on collaborative self-help efforts, it is important to note that the term self-help can more broadly refer to any self-directed undertaking aimed at personal improvement. Mental health self-help initiatives typically focus on mental health promotion goals such as enhanced coping and progress toward recovery (Brown, Shepherd, Wituk, & Meissen, 2008). Collaborative mental health self-help efforts have become increasingly widespread over the years and, today, mental health self-help initiatives outnumber traditional mental health organizations in the United States (Goldstrom et al., 2006). This growth is due in large part to their low-cost, devoted supporters, and increased acceptance by mental health professionals. Although these initiatives vary widely, they all emphasize mutual support and typically maintain a self-help/mutual aid philosophy, which values (1) the promotion of inner strengths, (2) a reliance on helping each other, (3) a rejection of hierarchy, (4) sense of community, (5) empowerment and participation, (6) self-acceptance and openness (Riessman & Carroll, 1995).

CROs are a specific kind of mental health self-help initiative. They differ from self-help groups, coalitions, and businesses in that they are typically incorporated nonprofits that can receive grants and often have paid staff governed by a board of directors, all of whom have mental health problems. Although CROs collaborate with nonconsumers to varying degrees, control over the organization always remains in the hands of consumers. CROs pursue a variety of goals but one of the most common is fostering mutually supportive relationships between people with mental health problems. Frequently, CROs achieve this goal by operating a drop-in center, organizing recreational activities, and/or hosting support groups. Other popular organizational activities include performing community service, raising public awareness about mental health problems, advocacy work, member education, and fundraising (Brown, Shepherd, Wituk, & Meissen, 2007a; Trainor, Shepherd, Boydell, Leff, & Crawford, 1997). Although organizational pursuits vary widely, there are some guiding principles that unify CROs. They provide empowering roles for people with mental health problems, emphasize a respectful, accepting environment, and allow for self-initiated participation and decision making (Holter, Mowbray, Bellamy, MacFarlane, & Dukarski, 2004). In the literature, several terms have been used to refer CROs, including:

- Self-help agencies (e.g., Segal & Silverman, 2002)
- Consumer-run drop-in centers (e.g., Mowbray, Robinson, & Holter, 2002)
- Consumer/survivor initiatives (e.g., Nelson, Lord, & Ochocka, 2001).
- Consumer-operated self-help centers (e.g., Swarbrick, 2007)
- Peer-run organizations (e.g., Clay, 2005)
- Peer-run programs (e.g., Clay, Schell, Corrigan, & Ralph, 2005)
- Self-help programs (e.g., Chamberlin, Rogers, & Ellison, 1996)
- Consumer-delivered services (e.g., Salzer & Shear, 2002),
- Consumer-run services (e.g., Goldstrom et al., 2006).
- Consumer-operated services (e.g., Johnsen, Teague, & Herr, 2005)

History of CROs and Mental Health Care

Over the past century, mental health treatment has seen drastic transformations and today a new philosophy is emerging in community mental health called the empowerment/community integration paradigm (Nelson et al., 2001). This paradigm stands in stark contrast to previous mental health treatment approaches. One of the earliest approaches to mental health treatment was the medical/institutional paradigm, which became dominant in the 19th century. This paradigm emphasized the use of psychiatric hospitals constructed to treat patients who had little, if any, control in determining their treatment. During the 1960s, the community treatment/rehabilitation paradigm emerged, providing alternatives to institutionalization that included supportive housing, clubhouses, case management, and other services designed to provide clients life skills so they would require reduced amounts of professional care, especially hospitalization. Although a significant advance, a number of issues in the community treatment/rehabilitation paradigm remain, including a focus on individual deficits leading to continued stigma and an imbalance of control between professionals and consumers (Carling, 1995; Nelson et al., 2001). Studies have found that the community treatment/rehabilitation paradigm helped many people have a physical presence in the community while remaining socially and psychologically unintegrated (Mowbray, Greenfield, & Freddolino, 1992; Sherman, Frenkel, & Newman, 1986).

The empowerment community/integration paradigm is now emerging in response to many of the weaknesses inherent in the community treatment/rehabilitation paradigm. This new conceptualization of mental health treatment emphasizes the importance of community integration, where people are a valued part *of the community*, not just *in the community* (Nelson, Walsh-Bowers, & Hall, 1998). Rather than focusing on illness and psychosocial deficits, there is an emphasis on strengths, potential for growth, and recovery. The paradigm additionally emphasizes empowerment, where individuals actively participate in and gain control over their lives. Increasing both empowerment and community integration requires a change in the roles of both mental health consumers and professionals. People with mental health problems must play the role of citizen rather than patient and professionals must play the role of "resource collaborator" rather than "expert technician" (Constantino & Nelson, 1995). This philosophical shift toward autonomy and self-sufficiency in the treatment of mental health problems provides important support for the use of CROs, which have a rich history of their own.

The oldest consumer-run initiatives are international networks of self-help groups such as Recovery International, which started in 1937 and became fully consumer controlled in 1952 (Recovery International, 2009). GROW is another self-help group network that was founded in 1957 by consumers who developed their own 12-step program based on the Alcoholics Anonymous model. Through the "self-help revolution" (Norcross, 2000), numerous other groups have followed their footsteps, including Schizophrenics Anonymous, the Depression and Bipolar Support Alliance, and Emotions Anonymous. Randomized trials indicate mental health self-help groups can be effective (Bright, Baker, & Neimeyer, 1999; Chien, Chan, Morrissey, & Thompson, 2005; Chien, Chan, & Thompson, 2006; Chien, Thompson, & Norman, 2008). However, the evidence is not unequivocal and it is clear that not all self-help groups are effective (Pistrang, Barker, & Humphreys, 2008). More research is needed to understand the conditions under which self-help groups are effective. Regardless, self-help groups remain the most prevalent form of consumer-run initiative and serve as the foundation for the development of CROs, which use more complex organizational structures and typically require external funding (Goldstrom et al., 2006).

The mental health patient's liberation movement has also played an influential role in the development of CROs. The movement began in the 1970s after deinstitutionalization, when "ex-inmates" who fiercely rejected the professional mental health system began to organize, developing self-help initiatives and advocating for consumer rights (Chamberlin, 1977, 1990). The ideology promoted by these groups has gained increasingly mainstream acceptance and their work continues to influence consumer initiatives.

Along with the burgeoning interest in CROs among consumers, elements of the professional mental health system have embraced the use of consumer initiatives and promoted it as a means toward recovery (Solomon, 2004). Such support is well justified, as research suggests the use of mental health self-help can reduce the need for psychiatric hospitalization, thereby reducing taxpayer burden for the mental health system (Burti et al., 2005). Further, mental health self-help participation can improve medication compliance (Magura, Laudet, Mahmood, Rosenblum, & Knight, 2002). In addition to supporting the use of volunteer-driven consumer initiatives, the mental health system has also provided funding for the provision of consumer and family-run programs. Examples of consumer initiatives that use funding include consumer-run drop-in centers, crisis residential programs, certified peer specialist training programs, and consumer technical assistance centers. Along with other organizational pursuits, the CROs studied in this book all operate drop-in centers, which is the most common type of activity for CROs, with approximately 1,400 operating in the United States (Goldstrom et al., 2006).

Increased consumer participation in the public mental health system has accompanied the growth in consumer-delivered services. Consumer voice in the decision-making processes of professional mental health organizations is growing (Fisher & Spiro, 2010). Additionally, consumers are becoming increasingly involved in the development of their treatment plan (Nelson et al., 2001). Further, professional mental health organizations such as the Veterans Health Administration (2004) are frequently hiring consumers as service providers. Fueling growth in consumer hiring is the fact that services of peer support specialists are now Medicaid reimbursable in a number of states (Sabin & Daniels, 2003). Nevertheless, mental health professionals have less confidence in consumer-run programs as compared to professional services and fewer than half of professionals have ever made a referral to a consumer-run program (Hardiman, 2007).

Research on the Effectiveness of CROs

Evidence supporting the effectiveness of CROs is convincing. The strongest evidence comes from two randomized trials. Intent-to-treat analyses from the SAMHSA/CMHS Consumer-Operated Service Program multisite randomized trial indicate that random assignment to a CRO with a drop-in center significantly improved well being, with a moderate effect size of .39 (Teague et al., 2005). Another randomized trial found that consumers assigned to the CRO plus standard treatment condition showed greater improvements in personal empowerment, self-efficacy, and social integration, as compared to consumers in the standard treatment only condition (Segal et al., 2010). Findings from the Segal study also indicate individuals in the CRO plus standard treatment condition demonstrated greater declines in symptoms and hopelessness, as compared to the standard treatment only condition. Other evaluations of CROs are also positive. For example, research by Trainor et al. (1997) documented a 91% decline in the use of inpatient services after CRO participation began. In addition, the Trainor study found that, on average, people with psychiatric disabilities considered their organization the single most helpful component of the mental health system. Furthermore, Yanos, Primavera, & Knight (2001) found that participants involved in CROs had better social functioning and used more coping strategies than those involved only in traditional mental health services. Finally, in a longitudinal observational study of four CROs, Nelson et al. (2006) found that after 18 months, active participants experienced increased social support, improved quality of life, and decreased psychiatric hospitalization, whereas nonactive participants did not change on these outcomes.

Mowbray and Tan (1993) found that when compared to community mental health services, 77% of consumers perceived CROs more favorably. Frequently cited differences included having more freedom, more support and caring, and less structure. Consumers also reported having organizational control (87%), feeling accepted (99%), and coming to their CRO out of their own free will (98%). According to members, CRO involvement led to increases in volunteer work, paid employment, and school involvement, whereas decreasing institutionalization, substance abuse, and the use of professional mental health services (Mowbray and Tan 1993).

People with mental health problems appear to be eager to get involved in CROs. From 2000 to 2003, as the availability of funding for CROs in Kansas increased, the number of organizations increased 75% from 12 to 21 and the number of members involved increased 114% from 582 to 1,244 members (Center for Community Support & Research, 2003). CROs are also cost efficient because of their small budgets and reliance on voluntary leadership, operating on approximately $8 daily per person in Michigan (Holter & Mowbray, 2005) and $11.51 daily per person in Kansas (Brown et al., 2007a). In addition to their low cost in comparison to traditional mental health services, research indicates that CROs achieved 69% of goals they set (Brown et al., 2007a). This rate of organizational goal achievement suggests general organizational competence. Member perceptions of CRO environments are consistent with the self-help ideology of providing a supportive environment, opportunities for active involvement in the organization, and the encouragement of individual autonomy (Segal, Silverman, & Temkin, 1997). Considering the low cost of these organizations, their ability to operate effectively, the benefits of participation, and their popularity among people with mental health problems, CROs have the potential to become a major component of the mental health system.

Organizational Dynamics

The organizational dynamics of CROs are both unique and generic. Like other nonprofits, they experience problems with funding, competition, collaboration, bureaucracy, and leadership. They focus energy on managing resources, including finances, volunteers, staff, and a space for activities. Unlike other nonprofits, their unique position in the mental health system as an organization operated by people with mental health problems make some of these challenges particularly relevant.

This section on organizational dynamics first explores the consequences of different organizational structures. Next is a discussion of the organizational capacity needs for CROs. Third, factors that influence the use of CROs are discussed. The challenge of maintaining consistent funding support and avoiding cooptation is the fourth topic. Following is an examination of competitive and collaborative interorganizational relations for CROs. Finally, this section examines the use of shared leadership as an important strategy for organizational success.

Organizational Structure

The organizational structure of CROs typically fall in the middle of a continuum between unstructured grassroots associations operated by volunteers on one end (e.g., self-help groups) and formal nonprofit agencies operated by paid staff (e.g., Red Cross) on the other. It is important to understand the strengths and weaknesses of different organizational structures because the structure of a CRO typically evolves over time and needs to be strategically managed. As CROs grow, they are likely to face pressure to adopt a more formal organizational structure. However, adding organizational structure to manage growth can have devastating unintended consequences as the advantages of unstructured initiatives are lost (Smith, 2000).

Unstructured groups lack role differentiation, which enables informal, highly personalized interactions between group members that are typically warmer, more encouraging, and more accepting (Wuthnow, 1994). The consensus-driven decision making typically used by unstructured groups also helps to promote the investment and involvement of all participants. The lack of hierarchy and bureaucracy encourages mutual support, intimacy, and sharing (Smith, 2000). Relying exclusively on internal funding also ensures independent control over organizational activities and prevents cooptation by external funding agencies (Brown et al., 2007a).

Although small informal organizations manifest several characteristics that promote CRO success, developing organizational structure also has several advantages. Large organizational size and hierarchical role differentiation enables economies of scale, which are more efficient at the production of goods and the provision of services (Milofsky, 1988). Obtaining external funding allows CROs to pursue activities and programs that cannot be accomplished otherwise. The role specialization and clear chain of command that accompany a structured organization can help promote efficient, goal-focused interactions and rapid organizational decision making. Training and certification requirements help to ensure that paid staff members possess the skills necessary to fulfill role expectations. Although these characteristics of structured organizations are frequently necessary for CROs to become effective service providers, they can also weaken the effectiveness of mutual support, which thrives in unstructured settings. Furthermore, there is concern that paying consumers to help other consumers will reproduce power inequities that currently exist in the professional mental health system. Regardless, using consumers as service providers can help to address the poverty level conditions experienced by many mental health consumers and may help to build stronger therapeutic alliances (Solomon, 2004).

CROs frequently manifest some characteristics of both structured and unstructured organizations because they were founded by a small group of passionate but often inexperienced volunteers that exemplify unstructured grassroots associations and developed into more structured nonprofit organizations operated using a mixture of paid and volunteer support. If CROs begin to receive grant funding or reimbursement for services, they often struggle to maintain the advantages of an unstructured association while managing the unintended consequences of becoming a nonprofit with a budget and paid staff. CROs need adequate structure to be accountable without compromising the grassroots camaraderie and passion that inspires the organization.

Previous research on the goals of CROs in Kansas provides insight into where these organizations fall on the continuum between formal nonprofit organizations and informal grassroots associations (Brown et al., 2007a). With respect to funding, CROs resemble structured nonprofits in their reliance on grant funding to continue operations, whereas grassroots associations remain financially independent (Smith, 2000). Furthermore, CROs are similar to structured nonprofits in their focus on maintaining or increasing their days and hours of operation. Grassroots associations typically have more intermittent rather than continuous activity (Smith, 2000). CROs retain many characteristics of unstructured grassroots organizations, however. Their reliance of voluntarism remains substantial and most implement organizational strategies to increase the number of members contributing voluntary leadership. The internal focus of CROs on reducing social isolation among members and celebrating member accomplishments is further reflective of their grassroots nature (Brown et al., 2007a; Fischer, 1982).

Maintaining the atmosphere of an informal grassroots association is central to the success of CROs. The small size, minimal hierarchy, and informality of these unstructured organizations all promote the development of mutually supportive relationships based on equality. Increasing organizational size, hierarchy, and formality augment the development of impersonal and rigid relationships between members. CROs must avoid such an atmosphere in order to be successful in helping people develop new role relationships that promote personal growth. If hierarchical role relationships become established, they can permeate the entire setting, leaving most members at the bottom of the hierarchy. The inequitable relationships that form and their unsatisfactory nature can lead people to disengagement and feelings of inferiority.

Hierarchical structures with paid staff shift the burden of organizational management onto a select few members. CRO members who are not getting paid have little influence over the organization and quickly fall into the disengaged service recipient role. If this occurs, CROs become no different from the mental health organizations they were originally a reaction against. The same roles are played and the same helpless and isolated lifestyles will manifest among people with mental health problems.

In contrast, the small informal organization encourages roles of responsibility for everyone (Schoggen, 1989). Help is needed from everyone and a sense of ownership in the organization is shared by all. When people fill these empowering roles, their behaviors will change. They can begin to identify as useful people who can contribute.

Organizational Capacity Needs and Technical Assistance

As nonprofits operated by passionate but often inexperienced individuals, CROs frequently need to develop new organizational capacities in order to succeed as nonprofits. The organizational capacity needs of CROs are similar to those of other small nonprofits (Wituk, Vu, Brown, & Meissen, 2008). Organizational capacities essential to operating a nonprofit can be organized into four categories (1) technical (e.g., grant writing, quarterly reporting), (2) management (e.g., business management, staffing issues, conflict resolution), (3) adaptive (e.g., activity planning, strategic planning), and (4) leadership capacity (e.g., board development; Connolly & York, 2002). Research indicates CROs frequently need assistance in each of these areas and technical assistance providers can be a critical source of support (Van Tosh & del Vecchio, 2000). Some of the most common types of support provided to CROs include grant writing, quarterly reporting, board development, and business management (Wituk et al., 2008). Longitudinal analyses suggest needs related to organizational infrastructure, such as the development of a strong board of directors and the establishment of effective organizational policies, may increase as organizations mature. In contrast, needs for assistance with attracting new members and attaining nonprofit status are more likely to decline over time (Wituk et al., 2008).

Factors Influencing the Use of CROs

Growth in the power of the consumer movement stands as a critical factor promoting the use of CROs. However, several other factors are also important. CROs can provide participants with several benefits that professional services are less capable of providing. For example, CROs may provide friendships, empowering leadership roles, and spiritual inspiration. Participants who obtain these benefits are not only likely to continue participation but may also share their experiences with others who may decide to join. Through word of mouth, many self-help initiatives flourish.

Several factors also impede the use of CROs. The stigma and discrimination associated with psychiatric diagnoses inhibits participation from individuals who do not want to further identify and affiliate with their psychiatric diagnosis (Brown, 2009b). Some potential participants also view CRO participation as a sign of weakness and associate CROs with people who are overly emotional and sensitive. Furthermore, professionals sometimes view CROs with suspicion, unsure of whether participants provide sound advice. Groups that depend entirely on word of mouth may be isolated and liable to falter without external supports such as referrals from mental health professionals. Unresolved internal conflicts may also cause some members to discontinue participation or the entire initiative to disband (Mohr, 2004).

Funding Support and Avoiding Cooptation

CROs and other nonprofits that depend on external funding continually face the challenge of maintaining consistent funding without losing sight of the organization's original mission. To meet this challenge, CROs must find appropriate funding agencies who are interested in supporting their mission. Consistent funding can be particularly difficult to sustain because of rapid changes in government and foundation-funding priorities (Dees & Economy, 2001). A healthy collaborative relationship can be sustained if the needs of both the CRO and the funding agency can be met.

Funding agencies need to ensure the accountability of funding recipients, which allows the agencies to make informed decisions about how to effectively distribute their resources. Funding agencies typically establish accountability using grant requirements that mandate nonprofits to report on their execution of grant-related activities. Cumbersome or rigid requirements can conflict with the organizational mission and operational philosophy of the CROs. When CROs face this conflicting situation, they may have to make an uncomfortable choice in favor of either obtaining money or maintaining mission integrity. Rejecting grant requirements may lead to organizational dissolution, whereas accepting grant requirements may compromise the organizational mission and philosophy.

The imposition of grant requirements by a funding agency can erode the autonomy of any nonprofit and operate as a form of cooptation or coercive cooperation, especially if the nonprofit is heavily dependent on a single funding agency. The introduction of new grant requirements restricting the independent decision making of the organization can occur gradually over funding cycles or suddenly, in a major overhaul of grant requirements. If grant contracts prohibit established organizational activities or funding becomes contingent upon the completion of specific activities that compromise the nonprofit's philosophy, needs, goals, or methods, then cooptation has begun.

Cooptation has historically been a problem for CROs (Kasinsky, 1987). Avoiding it is important because consumer control is a central tenet of their operation and a large part of what promotes empowerment and recovery (Holter et al., 2004; Brown et al., 2008). Organizational control by consumers is required so that members can find roles in which they can pursue their ambitions and control their surroundings. The disempowered and subservient roles that result from cooptation resemble the same roles traditionally found by clients in the mental health system. Although coercive grant requirements are clearly problematic, funding agencies typically have no desire to control a CRO. Instead, funding agencies create grant requirements in an effort to ensure accountability and the effective allocation of resources. Thus, developing strategies to establish accountability without compromising the independence of consumer initiatives is an important policy issue for mental health systems to address.

One strategy that demonstrates promise in establishing accountability while maintaining consumer control is the use of goal tracking. The use of goal tracking allows organizations to provide individually defined, context appropriate markers of success while still enabling the objective tracking and reporting of organizational goal achievement. Developing concrete, objectively measurable goals that serve as milestones of progress toward the fulfillment of the organizational mission can also facilitate planning and create a shared understanding of the logic behind tasks (Bryson, 1995). Periodically conducting an audit of goal achievement can serve to establish organizational accountability while also providing the organization with corrective feedback on their progress (Kiresuk & Lund, 1978). Finally, the process of setting goals and tracking organizational progress can enhance organizational focus and achievement motivation (Rodgers & Hunter, 1991). The use of goal tracking among CROs has been successful in Kansas (Brown et al., 2007a) and may generally be an effective strategy for demonstrating the accountability of grant-funded consumer initiatives, especially when technical assistance is available to support the development of appropriate goals.

Interorganizational Relations

Success often requires CROs to compete with other community agencies for money and participants. Competition can particularly be a problem for CROs in rural areas, where the sparse population creates a small population for mental health services. Competition for participants may arise between CROs and mental health centers because both struggle to attract enough participants. Because mental health centers can bill for services that are similar to some of the activities of a CRO, there is a strong incentive for the mental health center to "compete" for participants that would otherwise receive this support from the CRO.

Through interorganizational collaboration, CROs and other nonprofits can gain resources, knowledge, and influence (Hardy, Phillips, & Lawrence, 2003). Research suggests CROs with more organizational connections have more financial resources, have more members, and organize more activities (Center for Community Support & Research, 2004). However, this study found no relation between organizational network size and recovery attributable to CRO participation. Thus, the benefits of interorganizational collaboration may be more important for CROs with an external focus on social change rather than inward focus on personal change.

System-level activities that influence the human service system, the broader community, and social policy are also more likely to require strong community relations and interorganizational collaborations. Popular system-level activities among CROs include public education about mental health problems, political advocacy, and community planning focused on improving supports and services available to mental health consumers (Janzen, Nelson, Trainor, & Ochocka, 2006). Research suggests CRO involvement in these system-level activities can be both effective in achieving system-level change and in enhancing the credibility, awareness, and respect for consumer voices in the community (Janzen et al., 2006).

Shared Leadership

Sharing leadership responsibilities has been successful in preventing burnout and improving the sustainability of self-help groups (Medvene, Volk, & Meissen, 1997; Wituk, Shepherd, Warren, & Meissen, 2002). It can also be helpful in achieving organizational goals (Brown, 2004). Such sharing of leadership responsibility also contributes to the well-being of the members who take on the leadership roles. Segal and Silverman (2002) found that CRO organizational involvement was the best predictor of personal empowerment and social functioning. Thus, one theory of how people benefit from CROs is that an organizationally empowering participation experience leads to personal empowerment. This explanation of how people benefit from CROs, along with numerous others, will be considered throughout this book, as described further in the next section.

Overview of the Book

The goal of this book is to develop a more refined understanding of how people benefit from CROs. To develop a more comprehensive conceptualization of CROs, I use the concept of roles, which serve to integrate structural and psychological perspectives. A role is a set of behavioral expectations describing how one person is supposed to interact with others in a given environment (Brown, 2009a; 2009b). For example, in the role of CRO transportation provider, one may expect to provide rides to the CRO. The book builds on this concept to develop a rich theoretical explanation of how people benefit from CROs called the role framework.

Chapter 2 reviews existing theoretical explanations of how people benefit from CROs, using the concept of roles to identify similarities and tie these disparate perspectives together. Perspectives explored include the recovery model, community integration, sense of community, behavior-setting theory, empowerment theory, the helper-therapy principle, experiential knowledge, social comparison theory, and social support theories. Building on this theoretical foundation through the unique application of identity theory (Burke, 2003; Stryker, 1980), the chapter concludes by describing an integrative preliminary framework explaining how people benefit from CROs.

Chapter 3 describes a study designed to refine the preliminary framework. In the study, 194 CRO members responded to focused questions about how CRO participation is beneficial. Coding the responses into categories led to the development of a relatively comprehensive list of the benefits of CRO participation. Using the categories as a guide, the preliminary model was refined so that it could integrate all categories into its structure, thereby creating a more comprehensive explanation of how people benefit from CROs that I call the role framework.

Chapter 4 describes the unique methodology used to further explore the role framework. Journalistic life history narratives and documentary photography were used to create an ethnographic look at life inside and outside the CRO. The chapter details the study setting, study sample, participant observation process, in-depth interviews, construction of life history narratives, and analysis of narratives.

Chapter 5 presents the colorful narratives of seven participants in one CRO. The narratives illustrate how the lives of participants have developed and how their involvement in the CRO has changed their life course. The chapter also provides a narrative describing life inside the local mental health system and a narrative specifically exploring the CRO being investigated.

Chapter 6 examines how the rich stories can be analyzed to provide insight into the role framework. Each narrative is individually analyzed with emphasis placed on how the narratives can and cannot be understood using the role framework. After the individual analyses, the chapter provides an integrative summary analysis of all narratives.

Chapter 7 examines the influence of organizational characteristics on role and relationship development. Specifically, the chapter examines the relation between organizational size and the development of leadership roles, based on predictions from behavior-setting theory and the role framework. These predictions are tested using data from 250 participants at 20 CROs in multilevel regression analyses. Results provide insight into how behavior-setting theory and the role framework inform one another to enhance understanding of CROs.

Chapter 8 presents results from a study examining how role and relationship development influences recovery. The study uses structural equation modeling to examine the relation between involvement in different organizational roles and recovery. Findings indicate that both socially supportive friendship roles and empowering leadership roles predict recovery. Discussion focuses on how CROs can promote the development of a socially supportive and empowering environment.

Finally, Chapter 9 concludes the book, providing some general insights into the recovery process. The chapter considers the book's implications for practice and future research directions that can further improve our understanding of how people benefit from CROs. Additionally, the conclusion reviews the strengths and weakness of the methods used to develop and test the role framework.

Chapter 2
Using Existing Theory to Build a Conceptual Framework of Consumer-Run Organizations

Abstract This chapter reviews existing theoretical explanations of how people benefit from mental health consumer-run organizations (CROs). I use the concept of roles to identify similarities and tie these disparate perspectives together. Consideration of the recovery model and community integration aids the conceptualization of CRO outcomes. Behavior-setting theory and empowerment theory enhance understanding of how different CRO setting characteristics influence participation and benefits. The helper-therapy principle, experiential knowledge, social comparison theory, and social support theories provide insight into the interpersonal processes within CROs that lead to participation benefits. Building on this theoretical foundation through the unique application of identity theory, the chapter concludes by describing an integrative preliminary framework explaining how people benefit from CROs.

A variety of theoretical frameworks can be used to understand different aspects of consumer-run organization (CRO) settings, processes, and outcomes. Developing a rich theoretical understanding of CROs can provide insight into (1) how CRO settings can be most effectively structured, (2) how mental health policy and professionals can effectively support CROs, (3) who is likely to benefit from CRO participation, and (4) how to design theoretically sound CRO evaluations. This chapter reviews the most common theories and concepts applied to CROs and other collaborative self-help efforts. To help integrate the various theoretical perspectives reviewed, they are organized into four categories (1) conceptualizations of CRO outcomes, (2) theories regarding how CRO setting characteristics influence individual outcomes, (3) explication of interpersonal processes that lead to participation benefits, and (4) frameworks that help to connect settings, interpersonal processes, and outcomes. Table 2.1 provides an overview of each theoretical perspective as it relates to CROs.

Recovery and community integration help to conceptualize the goals and outcomes of CROs. Behavior-setting theory, empowerment theory, and sense of community describe how CRO-setting characteristics influence interpersonal

Table 2.1 Overview of perspectives used to understand CROs

Theoretical perspective	Core insights
Content addressed: CRO outcomes	
Recovery	CROs can help people reach a point at which their knowledge and management of their diagnosis, their skills, and their values enable them to live a meaningful, satisfying life
Community integration	CRO participation contributes to (1) physical integration by involving self-initiated interaction in the community, (2) social integration by enhancing social networks, (3) psychological integration by encouraging camaraderie and group collaboration
Content addressed: CRO settings	
Sense of community	The interdependent, mutually supportive relationships at a CRO promote a sense of community and commitment
Behavior setting theory	Overpopulated CRO settings may have numerous capable leaders, whereas underpopulated settings may encourage a larger proportion of members to undertake empowering leadership roles
Empowerment theory	CROs promote individual empowerment by emphasizing self-determination and coping strategies. Member control of organizational activities, governance, and administration provides organizational empowerment. Organizing advocacy and public education efforts enhances community empowerment
Content addressed: interpersonal processes	
Helper therapy principle	Helping other CRO participants can provides helpers with a sense of self-efficacy, equality in giving and taking, improved interpersonal skills, and positive regard from help recipients
Experiential knowledge	CRO participants may be more capable of extending empathy, emotional support, and relevant coping strategies because their similar experiences give them accurate knowledge and a deep appreciation of what a person is going through
Social comparison theory	CRO participation may normalize psychiatric diagnoses (lateral comparisons), provide accomplished role models who effectively manage their mental health problems (upward comparisons), and downward comparisons to those who are worse off, which may enhance self-esteem and appreciation of current capabilities
Social support	From a stress-buffering perspective, CROs provide participants with social resources in times of need. Long-term relationships also provide direct benefits (main effects), including a sense of stability, purpose, belonging, security, and self-worth

(continued)

Table 2.1 (continued)

Theoretical perspective	Core insights
Content addressed: connects settings, interpersonal processes, and outcomes	
Identity theory	Roles available in CRO settings provide members with opportunities to develop new health-enhancing identities
Preliminary theoretical framework	CRO settings promote the development of help seeker and help provider roles, where participants develop new skills to meet role expectations and adopt empowering help provider role identities

processes and individual outcomes. The helper-therapy principle, experiential knowledge, social comparison theory, and social support theories help to explain how the interpersonal interactions within CRO settings lead to individual outcomes. Identity theory provides novel concepts not previously applied to CROs that help to relate setting-level characteristics to interpersonal processes and outcomes. I draw from the ideas of identity theory to introduce a preliminary theoretical framework that helps to tie setting level characteristics, interpersonal processes, and individual outcomes together and helps to integrate the other theoretical perspectives. The following sections explore each of these theories and concepts in more detail.

Part 1: Conceptualization of CRO Outcomes

1A. Recovery

The recovery model represents a shift in thinking about mental health that is closely related to the empowerment-community integration paradigm discussed in the previous chapter. The two perspectives are similar in their emphasis on self-direction, autonomy, community integration, potential for growth, and collaboration with professionals rather than expert/patient relationships (Shepherd, Boardman, & Slade, 2008). These core features are valued by proponents of the recovery model, but debate about the nature of recovery remains, and its conceptualization continues to evolve (Bellack, 2006).

One defining feature of the recovery model is that individuals in recovery decide for themselves what constitutes recovery by developing their own hopes, goals, and concept of a valued life (Thornton & Lucas, 2011). The emphasis on self-determination in defining recovery stands in stark contrast to the biomedical model, where recovery represents an absence of impairments that deviate from normal biological functioning (Kendell, 1975). Self-determination is clearly important, but it can be counterproductive if individuals choose goals that compromise health. Thus, the recovery model is likely to be more effective if it also includes an explicit valuation of goals that promote human flourishing (Thornton & Lucas, 2011).

"Mental health recovery" also refers to individuals reaching a point at which their knowledge and management of their symptoms, their skills and values, their use of helping modalities, and their feelings about their life, together enable them to live a meaningful, satisfying life (Anthony, 1993). Recovery can be conceptualized as a combination of hope, self-responsibility, overcoming mental health problems, and moving past symptoms to cultivate a rewarding life (Deegan, 1988; Noordsy et al., 2002).

The self-determined nature of both CROs and CRO participation is consonant with the recovery model. As such, participation in a CRO can be a powerful part of one's path toward recovery. CROs help people build capacity and learn skills to overcome stressors and recover wellness. CROs can foster active coping and encourage taking responsibility for the consequences of one's actions, future, and well-being. By developing new capacities, framing new goals, and ascribing new meaning to old experiences, participants can create new states of wellness with renewed hope for the future. These all contribute to recovery. Thus, the concept of mental health recovery does not explain why or how CROs benefit people. Instead, it highlights the larger picture that CROs contribute to: helping people with mental health problems improve and refashion their lives in an adaptive response to mental health problems. This book seeks to develop a framework that can provide a more fine-grained understanding of how CRO participation promotes recovery.

1B. Community Integration

Community integration provides a different framework for understanding the many different ways individuals can benefit from CRO participation. Participating in a community is both a right (according to the 1990 Americans with Disabilities Act and the 1999 Supreme Court Olmstead decision) and an avenue to psychological and social benefits. Wong and Solomon (2002) thoughtfully define the interrelated physical, social, and psychological components of community integration. "Physical integration refers to the extent to which an individual spends time, participates in activities, and uses goods and services in the community outside his/her home or facility in a self-initiated manner" (Wong & Solomon, 2002, p. 18). Whenever individuals participate in a CRO, they do all of these. Thus, physical community integration is inherent in the act of CRO participation. The more someone replaces time spent in isolation with time spent involved in a CRO, the more physically integrated that person becomes into his/her community.

"Social integration has two subdimensions – an interactional dimension and a social network dimension. [The] interactional dimension refers to the extent to which an individual engages in social interactions with community members that are culturally normative both in quantity and quality, and that take place within normative contexts" (Wong & Solomon, 2002, p. 18). Again, CRO participation inherently involves social interactions with community members. CRO interactions are normative in the sense that participants voluntarily meet new people, share stories and discuss issues, solve problems, and take on leadership roles – activities common throughout community-based organizations. At the same time, CRO interactions are also often nonnormative in that participants interact only with other mental health consumers. This interaction may be helpful as participants share experiential knowledge in coping with mental health problems (Borkman, 1999), typically creating an understanding, accepting, and supportive environment where participants have a great deal in common. Thus, CROs facilitate social integration into the community of mental health consumers. However, socializing *only* with other consumers or CRO participants may limit a person's community integration.

"[The] social network dimension refers to the extent to which an individual's social network reflects adequate size and multiplicity of social roles, and the degree to which social relationships reflect positive support and reciprocity, as opposed to stress and dependency" (Wong & Solomon, 2002, p. 19). CRO participation leads to the development of a new social network full of mutually supportive roles. The more involved participants become, the larger and richer their social network will grow. Dependency roles do not typically develop because CRO participants act as both help providers and help seekers. The voluntary nature of CRO roles and relationships allows people to disengage from relationships in which stress outweighs the positive support received. Thus, CRO participation can dramatically enhance participants' social integration.

1C. Sense of Community/Psychological Integration

"Psychological integration refers to the extent to which an individual perceives membership in his/her community, expresses an emotional connection with neighbors, and believes in his/her ability to fulfill needs through neighbors, while exercising influence in the community," (Wong & Solomon, 2002, p. 19). This definition of psychological integration is very similar to the definition of psychological sense of community provided by McMillian and Chavis (1986). When interdependent, mutually supportive relationships form (at a CRO or elsewhere), a sense of community develops. People become attached and committed to the setting. They further invest themselves into the initiative, contributing to it and receiving many benefits from it.

Forming a sense of community is important to CRO settings because it promotes empowerment and catalyzes increased and sustained participation (Chavis & Wandersman, 1990; McMillian, Florin, Stevenson, Kerman, & Mitchell, 1995). Furthermore, a sense of belonging is a highly valued outcome of participation. A shared sense of community is catalyzed in many CROs by the shared "experiential knowledge" of members in a self-help initiative possess (Borkman, 1999). In a beneficial spiral, the warm accepting atmosphere inherent to settings with a strong sense of community is rewarding in itself, and is critical to the development of roles and relationships where participants exchange and sustain mutual emotional support. Having a place where people trust and support each other helps individuals gain confidence to take on new roles that are unfamiliar, exciting, and healthy. Settings rich with encouragement and acceptance allow people to take needed risks without the fear of social criticism. The trusting bonds enable communication around difficult issues and work as a healing mechanism (Gidron & Chesler, 1994).

Furthermore, developing a sense of community at a CRO can facilitate community attachment with other territorial (e.g., neighborhood) and relational (e.g., church) communities (Heller, 1989; McMillan & Chavis, 1986, Unger & Wandersman, 1985), thereby improving community integration. Research suggests that CRO participants are in fact involved in their communities; over 90% take part in at least one community activity outside of their CRO (Chamberlin et al., 1996).

In summary, the physical, social, and psychological aspects of community integration are important outcomes that CRO participation can promote, enhanced by the development of a sense of community. All fit with the larger conceptualization of recovery among people with mental health problems. Several other setting characteristics are also important determinants of positive CRO participation outcomes, including empowerment theory and behavior-setting theory. The next section discusses these, beginning with behavior-setting theory, which is useful in understanding how the CRO under- or overpopulation influences individual outcomes.

Part 2: Setting Characteristic Theories

2A. Behavior-Setting Theory

Behavior setting is a small social system defined by its standing pattern of behavior and occurring within particular temporal and spatial boundaries (Barker 1968). Established patterns of behavior guide the interactions among the setting's various participants. CROs are behavior settings that attempt to establish a mutually supportive pattern of behavior, where participants act as both help seekers and help providers, bounded temporally by their meeting hours and spatially by their meeting location.

For behavior settings to operate properly, the individual inhabitants that create the standing patterns of behavior need to be present. In behavior-setting theory, participants are essential to creating the standing patterns of behavior, but individuals are considered relatively interchangeable because similar interactions occur regardless of who occupies the setting. Assuming participants are equally effective at seeking and providing help, a CRO setting will produce a similar pattern of mutually supportive exchanges regardless of who participates.

One critical factor in determining how individuals experience a given behavior setting is whether it is under- or overpopulated. An *under* populated behavior setting has more roles than members, making every member essential (Barker, 1968; Schoggen, 1989) and requiring that some members occupy more than one role. In this environment, there are many opportunities to develop new skills, and all available resources are used. For example, rather than screening out less-adequate participants from leadership roles through "vetoing circuits," underpopulated settings develop "deviation-countering circuits" that help people learn the correct behavior and successfully perform the needed role (Schoggen 1989). However, if the setting is too underpopulated, members may become overextended and burn out.

In contrast, *over*populated settings have more interested participants than roles available. Therefore, such settings develop dynamics that select only the members perceived to be most capable to fill leadership roles, excluding other less-capable members. This process of exclusion within an overpopulated setting is called a "vetoing circuit." Both over- and underpopulation have important implications for individuals' experiences in that setting.

Research suggests that a strong leadership base is essential for effective CRO operation (Kaufmann, Ward-Colasante, & Farmer, 1993). Overpopulated CROs may be able to select only the strongest leaders and exclude weaker candidates. The competition can help CROs to operate effectively by putting the most capable leaders at the helm.

However, this exclusion of some members from leadership roles also may be problematic. Previous research indicates that involvement in organizational planning and decision making is an important predictor of participation benefits (Segal & Silverman, 2002). If there are a limited number of leadership roles, then overpopulated settings may confer less benefit on large proportions its participants. Instead, underpopulated settings may be more individually beneficial because all members are needed and encouraged to take on leadership roles. Furthermore, the idea that only some members are suitable for leadership contradicts the self-help ideals of minimal hierarchy and shared decision making (Riessman & Carroll, 1995).

Yet in any setting, participants gravitate to certain roles and avoid others depending on factors such as temperament, skill set, judgments of others, and opportunity. In overpopulated settings, involving everyone in planning and decision making can be slow and cumbersome. As groups grow, more participants are excluded from leadership roles since they are limited in number (Brown, Shepherd, Wituk, & Meissen, 2007b). However, exclusion from leadership roles may not be particularly problematic, as participants can still benefit from the mutually supportive exchanges that occur in nonleadership positions (Brown, Shepherd, Merkle, Wituk, & Meissen, 2008). These challenges of balancing leadership involvement with equality and effective operations are an important consideration for any CRO.

2B. Empowerment Theory

Like behavior-setting theory, empowerment theory provides insight into how setting characteristics contribute to outcomes. In this case, an empowering environment promotes individual empowerment and other benefits. Empowerment as a values framework recognizes that consumers have the right to gain control over their lives, make informed decisions about how they will use mental health services and take actions on their own behalf (Dickerson, 1998). As a process, empowerment involves developing skills and acquiring information to enhance self-determination. Environments facilitate this process when they value consumers' recovery and readily offer opportunities to both develop skills and acquire valuable information. Empowerment is also an important outcome fostered by CROs and positively related to indicators of physical and mental health (Israel, House, Schurman, Heaney, & Mero, 1989).

CROs are uniquely empowering because they are consumer driven. Furthermore, CROs are qualitatively different from professional mental health services in that CRO participants not only receive help but also provide it as well. Professionally delivered mental health services may provide excellent support, but even the most client-centered systems do not provide participants (clients) the benefits of helping others (see helper therapy principle, next section). The emphasis of CROs on building capacity to help oneself and others promotes empowerment (Trainor et al., 1997).

Thus, CRO participation leads to empowerment at the individual, organizational, and community levels (Segal, Silverman, & Temkin, 1993). CROs promote individual empowerment by helping members obtain needed resources, develop skills needed to take initiative in directing their own lives, and to become socially engaged. This is reinforced at the organizational level, in that CRO members control the activities that are pursued, their governance, and their administration. At the community level, many CRO settings encourage participant involvement in social change and policy making by organizing advocacy and public education efforts.

Thus, CRO settings often manifest key characteristics of empowering community settings, including: "(a) a belief system that inspires growth, is strengths-based, and is focused beyond the self; (b) an opportunity role structure that is pervasive, highly accessible, and multifunctional; (c) a support system that is encompassing, peer-based, and provides a sense of community; and (d) leadership that is inspiring, talented, shared, and committed to both setting and members" (Maton & Salem, 1995, p. 631). The sense of control and ownership that individuals can gain when participating in a CRO can transfer into a sense of personal and community-level empowerment (Schulz, Israel, Zimmerman, & Checkoway, 1995; Zimmerman & Rappaport, 1988). Furthermore, involvement in empowering leadership roles is an important predictor of personal empowerment and social functioning (Segal & Silverman, 2002).

Empowerment, sense of community, and behavior-setting theory all provide insight into how setting-level characteristics influence individual outcomes. The next sections describe how interpersonal processes in CRO settings help create these setting characteristics and contribute to individual outcomes. Specifically, the helper therapy principle, experiential knowledge, social comparison theory, and social support theories all help to explain how the interpersonal interactions that occur during CRO participation are beneficial.

Part 3: Interpersonal Processes Within CROs

3A. The Helper-Therapy Principle

The helper-therapy principle states that providing help can be more therapeutic than receiving help (Riessman, 1965). Research has demonstrated that helping others can improve self-concept, increase energy levels, and improve physical health (Luks, 1991). CROs provide many opportunities to help others in a mutually supportive environment. For example, participants help each other by providing emotional support, acceptance, and ideas about how to solve personal problems. Additionally, people in a CRO leadership role can help others by accomplishing organizational tasks that are beneficial to everyone. Such helping roles are especially valuable to people with mental health problems because psychiatric symptoms and the common consequences of severe mental illness (such as poverty, stigma, and discrimination) can reduce one's opportunities to make valuable contributions to others, such as through work, parenting, or civic leadership.

Skovholt (1974) theorized four benefits from helping others. One is an increased sense of competence or self-efficacy, which can occur when people successfully help others. For example, CRO participants may find that sharing one's own experiences and coping strategies gives other participants helpful ideas. This reinforces a positive self-assessment of those experiences while also creating the rewarding experience of being valued by someone else. Second, Skovholt theorized that helping others promotes a sense of equality in one's relationships, which can help consumers become independent, self-supporting adults, who contribute as much as they consume. A third benefit of helping is that it can promote learning and the acquisition of personally useful knowledge. In a CRO, people can apply their existing experience and knowledge in new ways, exercise problem-solving skills, expand their thinking about common challenges, and improve their interpersonal skills through helping others. Fourth, the helper role often leads to appreciation and social approval from the person receiving help and other peers. This positive regard can provide the helper with a sense of importance, usefulness, and satisfaction.

3B. Experiential Knowledge

Experiential knowledge refers to the insights, information, and skills that one develops through coping with life challenges. When people share a particular life challenge, experiential knowledge can help them relate to one another and provide appropriate support (Borkman, 1999). This shared experience is particularly powerful in a CRO because the prejudice associated with mental illness often sets consumers apart from others. Experiences with psychiatric hospitalization, medications, hallucinations, suicidal ideation, and other symptoms are not only hard to fathom but also often frightening. Friends, family, and even professional providers who have not had such experiences may therefore shy away from understanding these experiences, often by discouraging discussion of them and the feelings they provoke, changing the subject, or encouraging cheerfulness in spite of trauma (Coates & Winston, 1983; Dunkel-Schetter, 1984; Helgeson & Gottlieb, 2000). Such responses can frustrate and belittle people struggling to deal with mental illness.

Therefore, the shared experience with mental health problems among CRO participants frequently acts as a key bonding point in the development of supportive relationships. This commonality can engender trust and a feeling of acceptance. Numerous studies have demonstrated the emotional benefits of sharing experiences with others who have faced similar hardships (Helgeson & Gottlieb, 2000), including validation, normalization of the experience, a reduction in social and emotional isolation, and a sense of belonging (Cowan & Cowan, 1986; Lieberman, 1993; Rosenberg, 1984; Toseland & Rossiter, 1989).

Additionally, people who have also "been there" are often better prepared to provide appropriate support to each other by virtue of the (often hard-won) expertise and understanding that these experiences convey (Helgeson & Gottlieb, 2000). For example, mental health consumers may be more capable of extending empathy and emotional support to other mental health consumers because their similar experiences give them accurate knowledge and a deep appreciation of what a person is going through. By dealing with their own problems, CRO participants may also have developed coping and problem-solving strategies that can be useful to others facing similar challenges (Borkman, 1999). Their experiences may have taught them certain information, coping strategies, or tips that can save others from having to learn through trial and error. Thus, the exchange of emotional and informational support in a CRO, informed by experiential knowledge, can be invaluable.

3C. Social Comparison Theory

In CROs, participants' shared experiences enable several types of meaningful social comparison (Festinger, 1954). Lateral (peer) comparisons may serve to normalize and contextualize a person's experiences within the particular challenges shared by the group. For example, having a psychiatric diagnosis or caring for someone who does is often isolating because others cannot relate to the challenge. Discussing hopes, fears, stories, and meanings in a CRO setting can help people realize they are not alone in their struggle or abnormal in their reactions (Coates & Winston, 1983).

Second, CRO leaders are often charismatic and accomplished people despite the serious challenges posed by their mental health problems. Other members can make *upward* social comparisons to these people, viewing them as role models (Helgeson

& Mickelson, 1995). Their success may help raise the expectations, dreams, and motivation of CRO participants. If such participants can also identify with these leaders, socially valued roles may become a new possibility in their minds, perhaps replacing assumptions of isolation and dependency. Such upward comparisons may inspire hope and the pursuit of new life-enhancing roles. However, social comparison theory also cautions that the benefits of upward comparisons can be compromised if the more-accomplished person is seen as a rare, unattainable exception or too dissimilar from the upward-looking members (Suls, Martin, & Wheeler, 2002).

Every CRO has members with a variety of capabilities. Just as upward comparisons with the leaders are possible, so are downward comparisons with people in worse situations. Comparing oneself to others who are "worse off" may boost self-esteem by helping people appreciate what they do have (Wills, 1981). Downward comparisons also sometimes help people persevere in their coping (Taylor, 1983). CRO participants sometimes report that hearing other participants' more harrowing stories helps to put their challenges in perspective and increases their resolve (Lucksted, Stewart, & Forbes, 2008).

However, both upward and downward social comparisons are also potentially detrimental. Downward comparisons may lower expectations or contribute to demoralization, while upward comparisons may make people feel inferior (Helgeson & Gottlieb, 2000). How social comparisons play out in CROs is poorly understood and further research is needed.

3D. Social Support Theories

Social relationships are widely regarded as critical determinants of physical and mental health (Berkman, Glass, Brissette, & Seeman, 2000). Larger social networks among people with psychiatric diagnoses are linked to fewer psychiatric symptoms, improved quality of life, and higher self-esteem (Goldberg, Rollins, & Lehman, 2003). CROs improve social networks by providing participants with the opportunity to participate in shared activities that they self-organize and within which they may develop relationships that transcend those specific activities (Hardiman & Segal, 2003). Furthermore, research suggests that making new friends is the most frequently cited benefit of CRO participation (Mowbray & Tan, 1993). Relationships formed during CRO participation can be richly rewarding and therapeutic in themselves, and can also be valuable precursors to the development of relationships external to the CRO. Research by Trainor et al. (1997) supports the notion that CROs can help participants build networks in the broader community, with 60% of CRO participants indicating that contacts with nonconsumers increased as a result of their CRO involvement.

Social support, that is, the perception that one is part of a caring network of people who are helpful during difficult times (Cobb 1976), is widely recognized as an important determinant of mental health and a powerful motivation for CRO participation (Mowbray & Tan, 1993). However, *how* social support impacts mental health is extensively debated (Cohen, Gottlieb, & Underwood, 2000; Thoits, 1985). There are two prominent and competing models: the stress-buffering model and the main effects model. The *stress-buffering* perspective argues that social support mediates the relationship between stress and health. Enhanced coping ability made possible through social support can buffer the negative influence of stressful experiences on mental health because the resources available from social support provide individuals with both confidence in their coping ability and real support in coping with imposed demands (Thoits, 1986). By maintaining long-term relationships in a CRO, people are able to draw on these social resources in times of need.

In contrast, the *main-effects* model of social support emphasizes the importance of social relationships in the direct production of positive affect and the reduction of psychological despair (Cohen, Gottlieb, & Underwood, 2000; Thoits, 1985). Such relationships provide people with a sense of predictability, stability, purpose, belonging, security, and self-worth (Hammer, 1981; Thoits, 1983; Wills, 1985). CROs also provide these direct positive effects through enjoyable social interactions, positive settings for fostering further social relationships, and affirming exchanges about problems and challenges. Thus, CROs embody both the stress-buffering and the main-effects models of how social support contributes to well-being.

Part 4: Roles and Identity Theory

Identity theory and the concept of *roles* have not been traditionally applied to CROs; however, they provide important insights into how people benefit from these organizations. The concept of roles is helpful in integrating setting-level theories with interpersonal processes and individual outcomes because it provides a unit of analysis that is meaningful both to understanding the demands of behavior settings and individual differences in the nature and consequences of CRO interactions. Although there is no consensus definition of a role in the literature, a role can be defined as a set of behavioral expectations describing how one person is supposed to interact with others in a given environment (Brown, 2009a; 2009b; Brown, Shepherd, Merkle, et al., 2008).

Several social science disciplines have used the concept of roles to understand human behavior, including sociology (Mead, 1934), psychology (Lewin, 1948), and anthropology (Linton, 1936). Several role-based theories have been developed, including role theory (Sarbin, 1966), social valorization theory (Flynn & Lemay, 1999), and identity theory (Stryker, 1980; Stryker & Burke, 2000). All of these theories are meritorious, but the ideas presented in this book draw heavily from identity theory, a conceptually rich theory that grows out of sociological social psychology.

Identity theory (Stryker, 1980; Stryker & Burke, 2000; Stryker & Serpe, 1994) provides insight into the cognitive and behavioral consequences of taking on new social roles within a CRO. The theory is rooted in symbolic interactionism, a broad theoretical perspective within sociology pioneered by Cooley (1902), James (1950/1890), and especially Mead (1934). Although a review of symbolic interactionism is beyond the scope of this work, the perspective provides numerous concepts that are useful in generating a fine-grained description of human interaction (Hewitt 2003). In symbolic interactionism, behavior is thought to be guided by an active construction of reality using subjective interpretations (symbols) of our interactions with the world. Through our regularized social interactions (i.e., our roles), we make sense of our selves. We look to our environment to understand how we should behave in these roles. Identity theory contends, "persons live their lives in relatively small and specialized networks of social relationships, through roles that support their participation in such networks" (Stryker & Burke, 2000, p. 285). A person can play multiple roles within one social network, such as the role of mother with her daughter and the role of wife with her husband.

Numerous roles exist in CROs. Two universally available roles are that of help seeker and help provider. These roles do not have strict expectations, but some general guidelines are clear. In help seeker roles, participants may be expected to share problems, listen to feedback, decide for themselves which advice is useful, and develop plans to overcome personal challenges. Those in help provider roles may be expected to provide empathy, share their own struggles with similar challenges, share problem-solving strategies that have worked, and accept others for who they are. CRO participants typically occupy both help seeker and help provider roles on a regular basis, sometimes during a single conversation. Well-run CROs maintain role structures that promote mutually supportive patterns of interaction and allow members to move easily between help seeker and help provider as their needs and the needs of others indicate.

The different CRO roles are important to consider because people use roles as basic conceptual tools in thinking about self: the roles that we play determine our identity, which in turn determines the roles that we play (Stryker & Burke, 2000). Because roles provide purpose, meaning, direction, and guidance to one's life, Thoits (1983) theorized that a greater number of roles leads to a stronger sense of meaningful, guided existence. Her research shows that people who possess numerous identities report significantly less psychological distress (Thoits, 1986).

If people with mental health problems have small social networks and few social roles, then the stigmatized role of "psychiatric patient" is likely to dominate their identity, providing little meaning or purpose in life. Participation in a CRO can mitigate this problem by providing members opportunities to form new social networks, thereby taking on new roles in life. At a CRO, members may play the role of help provider in addition to their more familiar role as help recipient. Other potential roles beyond member include that of friend, board member, and volunteer.

When a role associated with a social network position is played on a regular basis, it becomes internalized as a "role identity" and adopted as a component of the self (McCall & Simmons, 1978). In social interactions, individuals draw on the most appropriate role identities in a given situation to guide their behavior. When a particular role identity is activated it serves as an "identity standard" or set of meanings that represent an individual's current self-concept. People try to behave in a way that matches their identity standard and they continuously adjust their behavior in an attempt to receive feedback from others that verifies that identity standard (Burke, 1991). The process of continually modifying behavior in order to achieve congruence between the identity standard and feedback from the environment is known as the identity control system (Burke, 1991). In this system, the "comparator" (a cognitive process) determines the level of congruence between the social situation and the identity standard. Meaningful behavior is then used to alter the social situation in such a way that it will be more congruent with one's identity standard. It is through this feedback loop that role identities have a major influence on behavior.

If an individual is unable to create congruence between the identity standard and the social situation, then the individual will experience anxiety. Because of this need for congruence, role performance is critical. An individual must be adept at performing roles to receive feedback in congruence with his or her identity standard. Adopting a new role forces an individual to build a new skill set in order to adequately perform the role. When individuals adopt new roles at a CRO, they will have to learn new skills to meet role expectations. These new skills may transfer to other community settings, thereby contributing to community integration.

The identity-control system process of matching the social situation to the identity standard is conceptualized as the process of "identity verification" (Stets & Cast, 2007). While people attempt to match their behavior to their role identities, they also try to shape their environment in such a way that their behaviors will match the social situation. People go through a process of selective interaction in which they choose to interact with others who confirm their identities (Swann, 1987). People also avoid those who do not support these high-salience roles (Swann, Pelham, & Krull, 1989). When discrepancies exist between the group member's role and the meanings of self-identity, the group member is less satisfied with the role and the performance related to that role (Riley & Burke, 1995).

This process of self-verification and role negotiation may explain many behaviors within a CRO. Identity theory would predict that when individuals join a CRO, they will seek out roles congruent with their identity. If they see themselves as passive people who lack competence, then they will likely find roles in the organization where they have no responsibility and can simply show up and enjoy the company of others. If they see themselves as activists, then they may find roles in the organization where they can make public presentations to reduce stigma about mental illness. According to identity theory, if people enter roles that do not support their identity, then they will experience distress and change their behavior in an attempt to find roles supportive of their identity. If individuals cannot find a role at a CRO that is congruent with their identity, then they are liable to stop participating and search for identity verification elsewhere. This may explain why many people show up at a CRO only once and never get involved.

The self is composed of various role identities that exist in a hierarchy of salience (DeGarmo, 2010). For example, an individual may be a father first and a businessman second, or vice versa. The most salient identities are the most likely to be invoked across a variety of situations. "Identity salience refers to the likelihood that a person will enact a particular identity when given the opportunity to do so. Identity salience in turn influences the actual enactment of social roles: the higher the salience of a particular identity, the more time and effort one will invest in its enactment, the more one will attempt to perform well, the more one's self-esteem will depend on that identity, and the more one's identity performance will reflect generally shared values and norms" (Thoits & Virshup, 1997, p. 112–113).

Identity salience is critical in determining how much a given role identity will influence behavior. The salience of an identity is hypothesized to depend upon identity commitment, which is both the number and the strength of relationships associated with a given role identity (Stryker, 1968). If an individual becomes involved in a CRO on a regular basis, then the role identities associated with CRO participation will move up the hierarchy of salience and begin to play a major role in defining the individual's self-concept. As relationships at a CRO become more important to an individual, the role identities played at the CRO will become more important to that person. Whether good or bad, these highly salient identities will have a major impact on the individual outside of the CRO. If CRO participation facilitates the development of a new salience hierarchy, then this new identity structure will have ripple effects throughout the individual's life, potentially leading to positive outcomes.

Borkman (1999), in her study of self-help/mutual aid, describes individuals moving from an identity of victim, to one of survivor, and then to one of "thrivor." Although she does not apply identity theory to the personal transformation, it still serves as a good example of how identity may change as a result of participation in a CRO. At first, people may come to a CRO as victims who are vulnerable and needy. As victims, they lack confidence and do not link their actions to consequences. By interacting with more seasoned members, sharing experiences, and receiving encouragement from peers, these new participants can begin to gain hope and make sense of their problems. Over time, individuals may begin to play the role of helper more often, building more self-confidence and gaining a sense of mastery over their past experiences. After becoming skilled in playing the role of helper, individuals may become thrivors, developing an experiential authority and playing the role of group leader or advocate. If the role identity of helper or group leader becomes highly salient, then individuals may begin to seek verification of these identities elsewhere, looking for other leadership and helping roles in the community. In this sense, participation in a CRO has the potential to alter the identities of individuals, helping them become active participants in the community.

Part 5: The Preliminary Framework

Drawing from the previously discussed ideas of empowerment theory, sense of community, the helper-therapy principle, social support, and experiential knowledge, along with concepts from identity theory (Burke, Owens, Serpe, & Thoits, 2003;

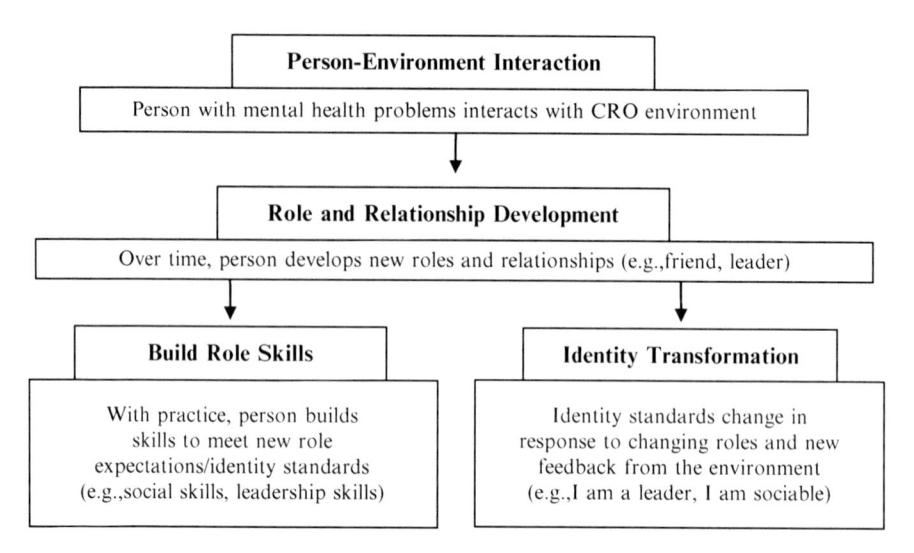

```
┌─────────────────────────────────────────────┐
│         Person-Environment Interaction       │
├─────────────────────────────────────────────┤
│ Person with mental health problems interacts │
│            with CRO environment              │
└─────────────────────────────────────────────┘
                      ↓
┌─────────────────────────────────────────────┐
│         Role and Relationship Development    │
├─────────────────────────────────────────────┤
│ Over time, person develops new roles and     │
│    relationships (e.g., friend, leader)      │
└─────────────────────────────────────────────┘
           ↓                        ↓
┌──────────────────────┐  ┌──────────────────────┐
│   Build Role Skills  │  │ Identity Transformation│
├──────────────────────┤  ├──────────────────────┤
│ With practice, person│  │ Identity standards   │
│ builds skills to meet│  │ change in response to│
│ new role expectations│  │ changing roles and   │
│ /identity standards  │  │ new feedback from the│
│ (e.g., social skills,│  │ environment (e.g., I │
│ leadership skills)   │  │ am a leader, I am    │
│                      │  │ sociable)            │
└──────────────────────┘  └──────────────────────┘
```

Fig. 2.1 The preliminary framework: how people can benefit from CROs

Stryker & Burke, 2000), the preliminary framework explains how people benefit from CRO participation (Brown, 2009a, 2009b). More specifically, the framework explains how the roles and relationships formed through CROs can lead to new skills and new identities. Fig. 2.1 illustrates the preliminary framework's four components: (a) person–environment interaction, (b) role and relationship development, (c) skill development, and (d) identity transformation (Brown, 2009a). The subsections below describe each component, followed by an explanation of how theoretical concepts presented earlier in this chapter relate to the preliminary framework.

Component One: Person–Environment Interaction

The first component of the framework describes how individual and environmental characteristics interact to shape the course of role and relationship development. Individual characteristics that are especially relevant to CROs include having mental health problems or caring for someone who does and being interested in interacting with similar others. Following is a discussion of several other individual characteristics that have been shown to influence participation in self-help settings and may be relevant in a CRO context.

Demographics. Several demographic characteristics may influence person–environment interactions and the subsequent development of roles and relationships. Previous research indicates older, more educated people were more likely to attend GROW groups (Luke, Roberts, & Rappaport, 1993). Minority status and gender have also been implicated as an important predictor of attendance

(Humphreys, Mavis, & Stofflemayr, 1991; Humphreys & Woods, 1994; Mankowski, Humphreys, & Moos, 2001). Differential effects by gender have been identified, with men benefiting more from the support provided by groups than women (Wandersman, Wandersman, & Kahn, 1980).

Level of social support. Lack of social support can make attendance in a CRO more attractive because CROs provide many opportunities to make friends. Indeed, Medvene et al. (1994) found that people with smaller social support networks were more interested in attending a self-help group. It may also be that socially isolated people can benefit more from CROs, as they have more to gain from the social support available at a CRO.

Similarity between self and group. Previous self-help group research suggests people prefer to be in groups with others who are culturally similar (Humphreys & Woods, 1994; Medvene, 1990). Similarity between self and group promotes mutual understanding, which may make the provision of social support more relevant and effective (Medvene, 1990). Intragroup diversity, however, is not necessarily problematic, as Luke et al. (1993) found mixed-gender groups promoted retention. However, feeling dissimilar from the rest of the group appears to be a barrier to engagement (Lee, 1988).

Environmental characteristics. One particularly important environmental characteristic is that CROs provide people who have mental health problems a setting that emphasizes mutually supportive roles rather than the unidirectional help-recipient roles that operate when interacting with mental health professionals. As further discussed in the section, "Relating the preliminary framework to other theoretical perspectives," environmental characteristics that influence person–environment interaction include the degree to which a CRO is empowering, has a sense of community, and is under- or overpopulated.

Identifying further individual and environmental characteristics that influence role and relationship development is a key research challenge facing CROs. Improved understanding of how the environment influences the interpersonal interaction process could foster the development of even more effective CRO environments that promote wellness-enhancing roles. Furthermore, understanding which individual characteristics influence the interaction process can help recruitment efforts target individuals who are most likely to benefit from participation and tailor skill-building programs within the setting.

Component Two: Role and Relationship Development

Whereas the first component focuses on characteristics of the person and environment (which influence role and relationship development), the second component focuses on describing the actual roles and relationships formed during CRO participation. A myriad of roles can develop during CRO participation, many of which are specific to a particular CRO. For example, a CRO may have an executive director, shift managers, and a board of directors. Listing the roles available in a setting and describing the expectations associated with each one can provide insight into the structure and pattern of interactions within that setting. The self-governed nature of CROs promotes the development of empowering leadership roles among participants because the continued functioning of the initiative depends on multiple members taking on leadership responsibilities (Maton & Salem, 1995). These roles have important consequences for their occupants, which are described in the next two sections.

Component Three: Build Role Skills

When CRO participants take on new roles, they may need to develop new skills in order to meet the new expectations. The third component focuses on understanding the skills that CRO participants develop in order to meet expectations. For example, success in the help provider role requires good listening skills; success in the help seeker role requires the humility to ask for help and the critical thinking skills to differentiate between good and bad advice. Leadership roles require participants to development several skills such as decision-making abilities. Skill development is one strategy people can use to meet the challenges and expectations of the roles they undertake. Their ability to meet role expectations enables the attainment of positive self-appraisals, positive emotions, and increased self-esteem.

Component Four: Identity Transformation

The fourth component focuses on understanding how the new role relationships in a CRO transform the identities of participants. Roles are fundamental determinants of self-concept because each role an individual inhabits on a regular basis becomes a component of that person's identity. These identities then provide a framework that guides role-specific interactions that the person has with others (Stryker & Burke, 2000). For example, people in the role of help provider may begin to see themselves as good listeners. Similarly, CRO participants who take on leadership roles may begin to see themselves as leaders. Once these identity transformations take place, CRO participants may become more likely to move into help provider or leadership roles in other community settings.

Identities shift as people embrace new role expectations and appraise their role performance. For example, a CRO participant in a leadership role may be expected to facilitate productive discussions during meetings. If the CRO participant successfully meets expectations, s/he will think of him/herself as a good discussion leader and may expand his/her behavior and identity in this role. In contrast, failure to lead productive discussions will lead to negative self-appraisals, negative emotions, and reduced self-esteem. This can spark behavioral changes to improve one's role performance, such as requesting coaching to improve facilitation skills. However, if failures continue, the person may escape the role expectations by giving up their role and identity. Thus, identity transformations are similar to skill development, in that they are a strategy people can use to maintain congruence between expectations and behavior.

Relating the Preliminary Explanatory Framework to Other Theoretical Perspectives

Several previously discussed theoretical perspectives are directly related to the preliminary framework, including sense of community, empowerment theory, behavior-setting theory, the helper therapy principle, experiential knowledge, social comparison theory, social support theories, and the recovery model. Within the person-environment component, sense of community operates as an important environmental characteristic of CRO settings that promotes the development of mutually supportive relationships. Similarly, an empowering environment is critical for CRO settings because it encourages participants to develop empowering leadership roles within the setting, thereby gaining greater control over their environment. When participants undertake empowering leadership roles, they can experience empowering identity transformations and begin to see themselves as leaders capable of controlling their lives and making important contributions to the community. Within behavior-setting theory, the concept of under- and overpopulation is a salient environmental characteristic for CROs that influences role and relationship development by pulling participants into leadership roles in underpopulated settings or excluding less-qualified participants from leadership roles in overpopulated settings. Experiential knowledge relates to the preliminary framework as an important individual characteristic that enhances person–environment interaction. The shared experience of coping with mental health problems helps individuals understand and identify with one another.

The consequences of role development described by the preliminary framework directly relate to two benefits of helper roles described by the helper therapy principle: an enhanced sense of self-efficacy and improved interpersonal skills (Skovholt, 1974). Through helper roles, people can build new skills such as interpersonal skills. Developing a sense of self-efficacy is a type of identity transformation that occurs when people become confident that they can meet the expectations associated with their helper role.

Among social support theories, the main effects model fit can be understood using the preliminary framework. CRO Participants can benefit directly from successful friendship roles because these roles help to boost self-esteem and provide participants with purposeful identities as important people embedded in the social network of the CRO.

Although not explicitly outlined in the role framework, both skill development and identity transformation are theorized to impact recovery. Skill development enables recovery because the new capacities can help people solve problems, achieve goals, and successfully manage life – challenges that would otherwise compromise quality of life. Identity transformation is fundamental to recovery for people who identify as helpless because they must begin to see themselves as capable individuals in order to have hope, personal responsibility for their own self-care, and confidence in their self-determined life choices.

Improving the Preliminary Theoretical Framework

Although many CROs developed without the use of formal theoretical frameworks, CRO leaders and allies can nevertheless refine their efforts through careful reflection on how their actions lead to desired outcomes. This chapter reviewed some of the most common theories applied to CROs and Table 2.1 provides a brief overview of each theoretical perspective. Although all have some empirical support, none has undergone extensive or rigorous testing in a CRO setting. It is likely that all are partially able to explain how people benefit from CROs. However, it is unclear which theories demonstrate the most promise and explanatory power. Subsequent chapters of this book seek to further develop the preliminary explanatory framework through empirical work, garnering insight into its explanatory power.

Chapter 3
Refining the Preliminary Framework to Create the Role Framework

Abstract This chapter describes a study designed to refine the preliminary framework presented in Chap. 2. In the study, 194 members from 20 consumer-run organizations (CROs) responded to focused questions about how CRO participation is beneficial. Coding the responses into categories led to the development of a relatively comprehensive list of CRO participation benefits. Using the categories as a guide, I refined the preliminary model so that it could integrate all categories into its structure, thereby creating a more comprehensive explanation of how people benefit from CROs. Specifically, the additional consideration of resource exchanges and self-appraisals allowed the model to account for all benefits described by participants. I call the revised model the role framework. The remaining chapters of this book further explore the utility of the role framework and provide preliminary tests of its predictions.

The previous chapter presented a preliminary theoretical framework explaining how people benefit from CROs by integrating numerous existing theoretical explanations. This chapter presents a study designed to refine the preliminary theoretical framework and enhance its ability to provide a more comprehensive understanding of the CRO participation benefits and the processes that enable each benefit. To ground theory development in empirical data, 194 CRO members from 20 CROs answered open-ended questions about personal changes that occurred as a result of their CRO involvement and which CRO participation experiences enabled personal change. Asking focused open-ended questions to a diverse group of CRO members provided insight into how participants generally think about the benefits of CRO participation (Iorio, 2004). Data analysis identified 18 personal change categories and 7 causes of personal change. These categories were integrated into the preliminary theoretical framework, which was then extended to accommodate all categories. Although inevitably tentative, the revised conceptualization, dubbed the "role framework" provides a more comprehensive understanding of the processes by which people can benefit from CRO participation.

Although not all-encompassing, the theoretical framework under study is more comprehensive than other theoretically driven explanations in the literature on CROs. The framework lacks its own empirical support, but it is transparently grounded in a large theoretical knowledge base with empirical support. The study presented in this chapter explores how the framework fits with the CRO participant's understanding of how involvement leads to personal changes. The empirical data gathered is compared to the preliminary framework in search of confirming and disconfirming evidence. Because the goal of the study is to develop rather than test the theory, the preliminary framework is considered a theoretical starting point in understanding data, rather than an ending point. As such, attempts to adjust the theoretical framework in light of disconfirming evidence are made.

Focused Questions Methodology

In order to understand the participant's perspective on how CROs are beneficial, 250 CRO members from 20 CROs were surveyed about their CRO participation experiences. Although a number of closed-ended questions were asked of participants, two open-ended questions are relevant for this study: (1) What personal changes have occurred as a result of your involvement here? and (2) What experiences did you have here that enabled personal change?

Study Setting

At the time of data collection, there were 20 CROs receiving grant funding from the Kansas Department of Social and Rehabilitation Services, Division of Mental Health and this study collected data from all of them. Researchers at Wichita State University's Center for Community Support and Research collected all data. This center also receives funding from the Kansas Department of Social and Rehabilitation Services to provide all CROs with technical assistance. CRO membership consisted solely of persons with a severe and persistent mental illness, as required by the Kansas Department of Social and Rehabilitation Services.

The 20 CROs in Kansas are diverse in terms of community size, operating budget, length of existence, and membership size. Some organizations exist in communities of less than 4,000 while others are in metropolitan areas greater than one million. The diversity in the number of members is just as broad, ranging from 9 to 171, with an average of 56 members. The average age of the organizations is 7 years, with one in operation for 26 years and two with 1 year of operation.

Operating budgets range from $5,600 to $132,000 with an average of $31,000. Although CROs frequently have multiple funding partners, including the local mental health center, businesses, and foundations, the primary funding agency for the 20 CROs in this study was the Kansas Department of Social and Rehabilitation

Services. The primary functions of CROs in Kansas are to maintain a drop-in center with activities that foster mutual support and provide leadership opportunities for the members. Additional organizational pursuits include increasing public awareness about mental health problems, fundraising, educational and training activities, and hosting support groups. There are several different ways members can get involved, such as volunteering for CRO activities, becoming a board member or hired staff, organizing activities, and helping maintain the facility.

Data Collection Procedure

Site visits were used to collect survey data during December 2003 and January 2004. Wichita State University's Internal Review Board approved study procedures prior to data collection. Researchers attempted to schedule site visits at times when the CROs would be heavily attended and CRO leaders encouraged attendance on the day of the site visit. During each data collection session, researchers described the purpose and goals of the visit. The method of survey administration depended on the needs of individual participants. Participants who felt comfortable independently completing the survey were allowed to do so. Participants who preferred an interview format were provided that option. In a few cases, researchers read each question to a group who then marked their answer on the survey form. Participants received $5.00 for completing the survey.

Study Sample

Of the 254 people eligible to complete the anonymous survey, only two people (1%) declined. Two surveys (1%) were omitted from the final data set due to obvious respondent error (i.e., marking all answers on the far right side of each page). Of the 250 survey respondents, 39 left both the personal change and experiences leading personal change questions blank. An additional 17 wrote N/A, none, or unsure on both the questions. The answers of the 194 (78%) remaining respondents were subject to coding analysis. There are several potential explanations as to why the questions were left blank. Some respondents may not have attributed personal changes to their CRO participation experience. Others may not fully understand how they have changed or know how to describe the changes that have occurred. Problems with reading comprehension and writing ability may also have inhibited individual ability to answer questions. Of the 250 respondents, 14% did not have a high school diploma or GED. Finally, survey fatigue may have prevented a response to questions. There were 73 closed-ended questions preceding the two open-ended questions.

The number of survey respondents from each CRO ranged from 2 to 32 and largely corresponded with the membership size of CRO. Frequency of participation was relatively high, with 21% participating every day, 59% participating several times a week, 13% participating once a week, 5% participating a couple of times per month, and 2% participating a few times a year. Length of participation was also relatively long, with 75% participating 1 year or more, 13% participating for about 6 months, 7% participating for a couple of months and 5% participating for a couple of weeks. Of those who have been participating for 1 year or more, the average length of participation was 5.2 years.

The 250 survey respondents ranged in age from 19 to 69 (mean 44) and 54% were female. With respect to race and ethnicity, 79% described themselves as White, 8% as Black, 8% as mixed, 3% as Hispanic, 2% as Native American, and 0.5% as Asian. Nearly half (46%) of the participants were single, 26% were divorced or separated, 23% were in a committed relationship, and 5% were widowed. In terms of highest education level, 9% graduated from college, 40% received some post-secondary education, 37% graduated from high school, and 14% had not graduated from high school.

Although it is impossible to know exactly how the sampled group differs from the population of CRO members, it is likely that this sample over represents those members most active in CROs (the regular attendees). CROs typically have a core group of members who participate on a regular basis. In addition to the core group is a larger group of people who sporadically attend. The convenience sampling method used is likely to have captured most of the core group of CRO members and a small proportion of the sporadic attendees. This bias was intended, as it facilitated a more representative sample of *active* CRO members. Studying these active members is advantageous because identity transformation is a relatively slow process that requires intensive involvement.

Data Analysis

I used QSR N6 (2002) qualitative data analysis software to facilitate data organization and analysis. The software allowed for open coding and text searching of all responses for keywords. Coding analysis of the answers of 194 respondents led to the creation of 15 categories describing personal changes, four categories describing the causes of personal change, and three dual categories that were both personal changes and causes of personal change. I conducted all the coding. Although the previously discussed theoretical framework inevitably influenced my understanding of the respondent's words, I created all categories in an attempt to describe themes that emerged from the words of informants. I used a constant comparative method of data analysis, where categories constantly evolved as new data were taken into consideration in coding. I frequently coded individual responses to questions into multiple change or experience categories, as informants often expressed multiple distinct concepts in one sentence. For example, I coded the response, "I have more friends now and higher self-esteem" into both a social network category and a self-esteem category.

Categories and Causes of Personal Change

Responses to the two questions were overwhelmingly positive. Four respondents listed negative interactions, but they did not form a coherent category. As such, they are not included in the results. There were also six responses left uncategorized because they were idiosyncratic and 18 responses left uncategorized because they did not make sense in the context of the question.

In coding analysis, the answers to the separate questions frequently overlapped, making it difficult to distinguish between the personal changes and the causes of personal change. For instance, one respondent described the experiences that led to personal changes by writing, "I made friends and became involved. It made me more confident in myself." In the second sentence, the respondent listed a personal change, rather than a cause of personal change, as the question asked. Even though it came from the question about causes of personal change, I coded it as a personal change because this change was not mentioned in the question about personal changes. Any time a causal statement was made, I coded the cause in the causes of personal change categories and I coded the effect in the personal change categories. As the analysis progressed, it became clear that some of personal changes were also being listed by respondents as causes of personal change. Social support, social networks, and helping others emerged as dual categories of personal change and causes of personal change.

Table 3.1 presents a list of all categories generated, along with the definition of each category, an example response, the number of respondents who mentioned each category, and the percentage of respondents who mentioned each category. The percentages are relatively small because respondents were not prompted to consider any particular category.

Table 3.1 Categories of personal change, causes of personal change, and dual categories ($N=194$)

	Number of respondents mentioning (%)
Personal change	
Self-esteem – feeling more valued, more confident, more pride e.g., "I feel better about myself as a result of a stigma-free environment"	39 (20)
Social skills – relationship skills, such as listening or communication e.g., "Socialize better, get along better with people"	37 (19)
Activity – becoming more active, spending less time at home e.g., "I get out more and am more involved"	28 (14)
Coping and problem solving – averting crises and reducing stress e.g., "I can deal with difficult situations better"	21 (11)
Outgoing – increased interest in and enjoyment of social interactions e.g., "I have been able to become more outgoing and talk to others more since I've been coming here"	15 (8)
Optimism – becoming more positive and looking forward to the future e.g., "I feel I have a future now and I look forward to it"	15 (8)

(continued)

Table 3.1 (continued)

	Number of respondents mentioning (%)
Belonging – feeling more connected to and accepted by others e.g., "Being a part of [CRO name] - cause I feel like I'm a part"	14 (7)
Conscientiousness – becoming more motivated and responsible e.g., "I am more likely to remember scheduled events in my life"	11 (6)
Independent – becoming better at managing life without a caretaker e.g., "I am involved in making decisions and that gave me confidence enough to live on my own and be by myself"	10 (5)
Paid employment – maintaining paid employment, frequently at the CRO e.g., "Since working here I've been able to buy my own townhouse and car"	9 (5)
Information – obtaining feedback and learning from others e.g., "Personal compliments or complaints from others let me know how I'm doing and what I need to work on"	8 (4)
Job skills – learning marketable skills, such as computer skills e.g., "I have become more competent on the computer writing grants and more confident giving input in group situations and being in charge of activities"	7 (4)
Less hospitalization – spending less time in a psychiatric hospital e.g., "I have been able to stay out of the state hospital better"	4 (2)
Generic improvement – unclassifiable overarching improvement e.g., "Everything is better"	11 (6)
Dual categories (emerged as both a personal change and a cause)	
Social network – meeting new people and making more friends e.g., "I have made more friends in Kansas than before I started coming to [CRO name]"	22 (11) – change 15 (8) – cause
Social support – having a caring place to exchange emotional support e.g., "I can come here when I need someone to talk to. There is someone here that will listen"	12 (6) – change 14 (7) – cause
Help provider – becoming an active contributor; being and feeling useful e.g., "Being on the board and having people depend on me"	18 (9) – change 12 (6) – cause
Causes of personal change	
Interpersonal interaction – interacting with others at the CRO, frequently in the context of recreational and work activities e.g., "I feel better about myself to socialize with people at night, otherwise I'd be at home watching TV"	54 (28)
Work – voluntary or paid involvement in organizational operations at the CRO, including both leadership and support roles e.g., "The joy of working with likeminded people to achieve long term goals"	37 (19)
Positive atmosphere – the organization is described using terms such as friendly, open, understanding, safe, and non-judgmental e.g., "Having people who understand what is going on with me and not put me down"	14 (7)
Recreation – involvement in any CRO recreational activity except socializing, which is categorized with interpersonal interaction e.g., "I have a chance to participate in activities and enjoy myself"	13 (7)

Integrating Categories to Create the Role Framework

If a comprehensive theoretical conceptualization is the goal, then the explanatory framework should account for all empirical categories. This section explores how the theoretical framework can account for the empirical categories generated by this study. Although data analysis proved useful in generating the categories a comprehensive framework needs to consider, data analysis could not provide insight into the relationship between personal changes and the causes of personal change. Relationships and causal connections that respondents made between categories were too scattered for themes to emerge. In the words of CRO participants, all of the personal changes are related to all of the causes of personal change. Although this reflects the interrelated nature of the different CRO participation experiences and personal changes occurring, it does not provide a parsimonious theoretical explanation of how people can benefit from CROs.

Considering the large number of categories, it appears as though there are innumerable ways in which CROs can be conceptualized. However, many of the categories are interrelated and maintain strong ties to the causes of personal change. Taking a step back from the data allows a larger process integrating the disparate categories to emerge.

The preliminary theoretical framework is useful in conceptualizing this larger process; however, some categories could not be easily incorporated into the original framework. These include *self-esteem, optimism, social support, paid employment, and information*. In order to incorporate these categories, I expanded the conceptual framework. The conceptual addition of resource exchange and self-appraisal components allows for their integration without compromising the cohesion of the framework. Further justification for the inclusion of these components, along with a more detailed explanation of their meaning, is provided in the following resource exchange and self-appraisal subsections, which are part of the larger explanation of the revised framework. The revised framework is dubbed the role framework. Its basic structure does not change throughout the rest of the book, although subsequent chapters provide additional insight into its utility.

Figure 3.1 illustrates the role framework and shows how the categories generated by short-answer questions fit into the framework. The process of fitting categories into framework components was driven primarily by logic rather than data, and a different perspective may have led to the placement of categories into different components. Each component of the role framework is described in its own subsection below, with an explanation of how the categories fit into and flesh out each component. In the narrative explanation, categories are *italicized*.

Person–Environment Interaction

People interact with CROs through *recreation* and *work*. *Recreation* varies from organization to organization but includes playing cards, pool, board games, puzzles, smoking cigarettes, ping-pong, crafts, cooking, gardening, cookouts,

```
┌─────────────────────────────────────┐
│     Person-Environment Interaction  │
└─────────────────────────────────────┘
┌─────────────────────────────────────────┐
│           Work; Recreation;             │
│ Interpersonal interaction; Positive atmosphere │
└─────────────────────────────────────────┘
                    ↓
┌─────────────────────────────────────┐
│    Role & Relationship Development  │
└─────────────────────────────────────┘
┌─────────────────────────────────────────────┐
│  Activity; Help provider; Social networks   │
└─────────────────────────────────────────────┘
    ↓           ↓            ↓           ↓
┌────────┐  ┌──────────┐  ┌────────┐  ┌──────────────┐
│Resource│  │Self-     │  │Build   │  │Identity      │
│Exchange│  │Appraisal │  │Role    │  │Transformation│
│        │  │          │  │Skills  │  │              │
├────────┤  ├──────────┤  ├────────┤  ├──────────────┤
│Social  │  │          │  │Social  │  │Outgoing      │
│support │  │Self-     │  │skills  │  │Conscientious │
│Informa-│  │esteem    │  │Coping  │  │Independent   │
│tion    │  │Optimism  │  │skills  │  │Belonging     │
│Paid em-│  │          │  │Job     │  │              │
│ployment│  │          │  │skills  │  │              │
└────────┘  └──────────┘  └────────┘  └──────────────┘
```

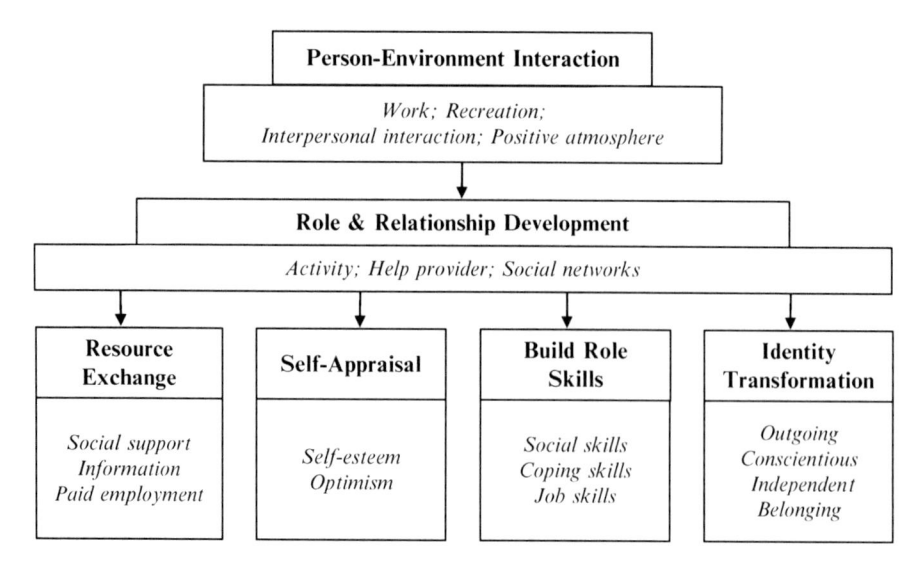

Fig. 3.1 The role frameworks explanation of how people can benefit from CROs

camping, shopping, and parties. *Work* takes a variety of forms, including writing grants, cleaning, building maintenance, planning/setting up activities, conducting volunteer work in the community, creating newsletters, making public presentations, recruiting members, recognizing volunteers with awards, completing quarterly reports, operating a warm line, providing transportation, purchasing supplies, and going to board meetings.

By participation in these *work* and *recreation* activities, people experience a wide variety of *interpersonal interactions*. Many respondents cited a *positive atmosphere* as an important environmental characteristic that promoted organizational involvement. Respondents described the CRO atmosphere using terms such as friendly, open, understanding, safe, and non-judgmental.

Role and Relationship Development

If people continue to interact in the CRO, new roles and relationships will develop and an individual's *social network* will expand. As long as the new roles and relationships continue, they will consume individual energy and people will experience increased *activity*. Keeping busy and engaged in these role relationships can add healthy levels of stress to a person's life, providing focus and purpose, while preventing aimless wandering and boredom (Thoits, 1985).

Both friendship and leadership roles can change the way CRO participants interact with others because they involve helping others. Several respondents mentioned the act of being a *help provider* as both an experience that led to personal changes and as a personal change in and of itself. This stands in stark contrast to the many dependency roles consumers typically play. In the professional mental health system, consumers receive a variety of government-funded services from therapists, case managers, attendant care workers, and doctors. Frequently, consumers live in a world where they do little for themselves or anyone else.

Resource Exchange

Embodied but not emphasized in identity theory is the fact that a resource exchange takes place when people engage in role-oriented behavior. Roles are defined and described by the reciprocal rights and obligations within a relationship (Thoits, 1985). In other words, roles consist of patterned interactions where people give what is expected of them (their obligations) and in turn receive what they expect (their rights). Drawing from the ideas of resource theory (Foa & Foa, 1974), these rights and obligations can be thought of as an exchange of resources. For example, in the role of *paid employee* people give their time and energy to the CRO in exchange for financial compensation. This role establishes an interdependent resource exchange, where the CRO benefits from the employee's services and the employee benefits from both the paychecks and the intrinsic rewards of being in a helper role.

Identity theory focuses on intrinsic rewards, such as positive self-appraisals, a sense of mastery or environmental control, and a sense of purpose in life (Thoits, 1985). While these benefits are certainly important, data from this study suggest that the resource exchanges themselves are important outcomes derived from CRO participation. Respondents discussed *paid employment* as an important personal change, rather than as an experience that led to change. Because CRO members often live on disability income alone, they live in relative poverty. Small amounts of income can help to solve problems, reduce stress, and provide everyday comforts.

Another resource exchanged during CRO participation is *social support*. CRO participants discussed the exchange of *social support* as both an important personal change and as a cause of personal change. Social support can be conceptualized as consisting of three categories – tangible (e.g., money, transportation), emotional (e.g., love, empathy), and informational (e.g., directions, service system knowledge) (Thoits, 1985). Social support at a CRO can take all of these different forms. When a CRO friend volunteers to baby-sit, tangible social support is being provided. Similar to the tangible support of *paid employment*, these exchanges can solve problems, reduce stress, and provide everyday comforts. The importance of informational support is reflected in the category *information*. Respondents frequently discussed the utility of the information obtained during their social interactions at the CRO. The feedback obtained can help people solve problems and understand different perspectives. Both receiving and especially giving support with a mental health self-help context predict improvements in social adjustment (Roberts et al., 1999).

Self-Appraisal

Self-appraisal is a key process in the previously discussed identity control system (Burke, 1991). In the identity control system, people give to the environment meaningful behavior in hopes of meeting the perceived expectations of the environment. If individuals perceive their behavior to be successful in meeting role expectations, then they will obtain positive self-appraisals and verify their identity standard. At times, the environment explicitly reflects positive appraisals but other times the actors must infer appraisals (Thoits, 1985).

For example, if a CRO member provides thanks after receiving a ride from a fellow CRO member, s/he is reflecting a positive appraisal to the person who provided a ride. As long as the ride provider interprets this reflected appraisal positively, s/he will receive positive self-regard for a job well done. If the ride recipient says only goodbye and not thank you, then appraisal must be inferred. If the ride provider perceives the ride recipient was dissatisfied with the ride, then positive self-appraisal will not occur. Perhaps the car is very dirty and the ride recipient was uncomfortable. In this case, a negative self-appraisal occurs as the ride provider has failed to fulfill role expectations. Sense of self-esteem is damaged if driver concludes s/he is not good at the role of ride provider, or more broadly, helpful friend.

This process of self-appraisal through social interaction is thought to be the primary mechanism by which people establish self-esteem (Thoits, 1985). Positive self-appraisal is synonymous with positive evaluations of one's overall worth, lovability, and importance. Whereas positive self-appraisal contributes to psychological well-being, negative self-appraisal contributes to anxiety and depression (Kaplan, 1980).

Any social interaction provides opportunities for people to develop roles that contribute to *self-esteem,* but CRO participation may be unique in that it promotes the development of helper roles. Numerous positive reflective appraisals are attained in helper roles, thereby encouraging positive self-appraisal and increasing self-esteem. Further, by consistently obtaining positive appraisals in a role, people can become *optimistic* about their ability to meet role expectations in the future and maintain the rewarding role relationships established at the CRO.

Building Role Skills

Over time, as CRO participants gain experience playing different roles, they develop the skills necessary to fulfill expectations in each of these roles. In helping others and learning how to fend for oneself outside of a dependency role, people learn *coping and problem-solving skills.* By the practice of solving your own problems and helping others solve their problems, *coping and problem solving skills* improve. In other roles, people build different skills. For example, in the role of friend people learn *social skills* by practicing communication, listening, and conflict resolution on a regular basis. In leadership roles, such as employee or volunteer, people learn *job skills.*

Identity Transformation

The development of an identity as an *independent* person may also result from the helper role because people give at least as much as they receive in a relationship. No longer are people eliciting pity and receiving help without giving back. By the formation of reciprocal relationships, CRO participants become needed. As such, they develop a sense of increased *independence* because they earn what they receive.

The adoption of leadership roles may lead CRO participants to identify as *conscientious*. For example, in roles such as board member, shift manager, or peer counseling coordinator, CRO members need to act *conscientiously* in order to meet the behavioral expectations associated with these roles.

Viewing oneself as more *outgoing* may result from playing the role of a friend. By spending more time socializing and developing social skills, individuals can begin to identify as *outgoing* people. Once people identity as outgoing, they may activate this expectation in multiple settings. The friendship and leadership roles may also contribute to a *sense of belonging*. Identifying oneself as a part of the CRO enhances commitment to the CRO and provides people with a comfortable safe haven when they have nowhere else to go.

Discussion

Based on the responses of 194 participants, the categories generated by this study provide a rich description of the types of experiences that CRO participants found beneficial and convey a clear sense of how CRO participants felt they benefitted from involvement. Furthermore, the categories serve as a relatively comprehensive list of CRO participation benefits and the participation experiences that lead to these benefits. This is a useful contribution to the literature on CROs, as these questions have not been addressed in existing research known to the author. Although the categories stand alone as useful information, they also facilitated the development of a comprehensive explanation of how people can benefit from CRO participation.

In this revised theoretical conceptualization (i.e., the role framework), the individual characteristics of CRO participants interact with the organizational context to determine the course of role and relationship development. Interpersonal interactions during the work and recreational activities of the CRO frequently lead to the development of friendship and leadership roles. Both are helper roles, which have distinctly different expectations from the dependency roles that consumers often occupy in the professional mental health system. CRO participants can obtain a variety of benefits when such helper roles are established. First, resource exchanges occur as a part of the regularized social interactions of role involvement. People give and receive tangible, emotional, and informational resources, which can help in coping with everyday challenges. These resource exchanges are guided by role expectations, which people attempt to fulfill in order to verify identity standards. If successful, people obtain positive self-appraisals, thereby enhancing self-esteem and emotional well-being. By practice, CRO participants become more adept at meeting their friendship and leadership role expectations. Coping skills, social skills, and job skills develop, enabling a mastery of role expectations. With new roles and accompanying skills established, people experience identity transformations and alter their self-descriptions. They may begin to see themselves as more independent, outgoing, and conscientious. Such skill developments and identity transformations may generalize outside the CRO as people begin to seek enactment of these new role identities in other contexts.

Connecting Framework Revisions to the Existing Literature

The role framework provides a more robust understanding of how people benefit from CROs. The added richness provided by the conceptual expansion enables additional connections to the existing explanations discussed in the previous chapter. Specifically, the role framework better captures processes discussed by the helper therapy principle, the stress buffering and main effect models of social support, social comparison theory, experiential knowledge, and the recovery model.

With respect to the helper therapy principle, two of the four benefits of helping described by Skovholt (1974) were captured by the preliminary framework: sense of self-efficacy and improved interpersonal skills. The new components in the revised framework relate to the other two benefits of helping described by Skovholt: equality in giving and taking and positive regard from help recipients. The sense of equality in giving and taking is related to the resource exchange component: as people in mutually supportive helper roles exchange resources, they develop a sense of equality in giving and taking. Positive regard from help recipients relates to the self-appraisal component: people in helper roles are likely to make positive self-appraisals because of the positive regard they receive from help recipients.

With regard to the social support theories, the stress-buffering model relates best to the resource exchange component: CRO participants who maintain socially supportive friendship roles can buffer stressful experiences by drawing upon their social support resources in times of need. The main effects model fit can also be better understood with the addition of the self-appraisal component. Participants can benefit directly from their friendship roles when they fulfill role expectations for being a good friend and thereby obtain positive appraisals.

New components of the theoretical framework also relate to social comparison theory, experiential knowledge, and recovery. Social comparison theory relates to the self-appraisal component. Members of a CRO social network make upward, downward, and lateral social comparisons that can influence their self-appraisals and role expectations as a person with mental health problems. Experiential knowledge and the resource exchange component relate to one another because experiential knowledge serves as a valuable resource that participants share during mutually supportive exchanges. Both the resource exchange component and the self-appraisal component relate to the recovery model. Resource exchanges enable acquisition of the support necessary to solve problems and cope with various stressors that hinder recovery. Self-appraisals are central to emotional health and a satisfying life, both of which are goals of recovery. Further, self-appraisals provide people with the confidence needed (or lack thereof) to address entrenched problems compromising their well-being and recovery (Corrigan et al., 2005).

Limitations and Future Research

The primary limitation of the role framework is its lack of empirical support. Although the planned data analysis intended to provide an understanding of how CRO participation experiences led to personal changes, consistent patterns connecting the participation experiences to the personal changes did not emerge. As such, only theory and logic were used to connect the personal change categories to the causes of personal change. Future research needs to explore whether the proposed connections between personal changes and the causes of personal change are consistent with the perspective of CRO participants. Additionally, since only one person coded the data, inter-rater reliability could not be calculated. Another limitation of the data analysis is that I used cross-sectional data to study a longitudinal phenomenon. Future research needs to study the benefits of CRO participation prospectively, thereby enabling a more reliable understanding of how the change processes unfold over time. Finally, quantitative studies that can rigorously test whether the proposed processes unfold as hypothesized need to be conducted before the role framework can be considered anything but tentative.

A second major weakness of this study is the fact that the revised theoretical model is derived post hoc from the data. A theoretical model that rests on data from one study is undoubtedly tentative. However, the model is rooted in both a large theoretical base and the data from this study. As a study intended to develop theory, it has been successful. New understandings of both the data and the theoretical literature have been generated and a theory with more promise has been developed.

Conclusions

The study presented in this chapter provides a tentative but promising explanation of the processes by which people can benefit from CRO participation. The role framework incorporates the ideas of several prominent explanations of how CRO participation is beneficial while maintaining a strong relationship with the CRO participant's perspective. The role framework stands as a promising step toward the development of a comprehensive understanding of how CROs are beneficial. This chapter concludes the explanation of the theoretical foundations and empirical research undertaken to develop the role framework. The remainder of the book continues to explore the utility of the role framework and test its predictions.

Chapter 4
Constructing Journalistic Life History Narratives to Explore the Role Framework

Abstract This chapter describes a unique methodology used to explore the utility of the role framework in conceptualizing how people benefit from mental health consumer-run organizations (CROs). The methodology is innovative in that it combines traditional ethnographic methods with the traditions of journalism to create compelling life history narratives. The narratives have strong didactic potential because they are accessible to lay audiences. Data collection consisted of participant observation, in-depth interviews, and documentary photography. The narratives provide an ethnographic look at the lived experience of having mental health problems, participating in a CRO, and making recovery progress. The chapter details the study setting, study sample, participant observation process, in-depth interviews, construction of life history narratives, and analysis of narratives.

The previous chapter explored the comprehensiveness of the theoretical framework. After making theoretical extensions, the role framework was flexible enough to capture the personal changes and causes of personal change described by 194 CRO participants. This chapter describes the innovative methods used for a follow-up study designed to provide an in-depth understanding of the change processes experienced by a small number of CRO members. The follow-up study used fewer informants than the previous chapter's analysis of responses to focused questions. However, each informant was studied in more depth, thereby providing a richer, more contextualized understanding of the change processes experienced during CRO participation.

The current study used data from participant observation and in-depth minimally structured interviews to produce life history narratives. The narratives detail the lives of seven participants at one CRO. The use of prolonged engagement, persistent observation, and triangulation increases the credibility of the findings (Lincoln & Guba, 1986). Additionally, the use of thick descriptive data increases the transferability of the findings because readers can make judgments about the degree of fit or similarity between the context studied and the context where findings might be applied (Lincoln & Guba, 1986). The analysis of informant responses to focused questions was limited by its inability to show how CRO participation experiences relate to personal changes. The use of life history narratives overcomes that limitation. By careful analysis of life histories, connections between life experience and personal change can be made.

The methods of the follow-up study are described in detail in this chapter for two reasons. First, thorough consideration of the methods is critical for the reader to judge the value of the narratives presented in Chap. 5, along with the analysis of narratives presented in Chap. 6. Second, the integration of journalistic and ethnographic methods used in this study is innovative. The integration of journalistic techniques into the creation of life history narratives helps to produce more compelling narratives that can engage a broader audience. Qualitative researchers interested in conducting similar studies will find the in-depth discussion of methods helpful. Details on the methods of this study are presented in the following eight sections: (a) conceptual and epistemological foundations of narrative, (b) the integration of journalism and ethnographic research, (c) visual storytelling, (d) study setting, (e) study sample, (f) participant observation, (g) minimally structured interviews, (h) life history construction, (i) analysis of narratives, and (j) sharing narratives.

Conceptual and Epistemological Foundations of Narrative

Narratives maintain several different conceptual foundations and purposes in the social sciences. For example, Bruner (1987) argued that narratives are the primary means by which humans understand and describe life. As a root metaphor for psychology, narratives serve to both guide our own behavior and understand the behavior of others (Sarbin, 1986). Narratives are also considered fundamental organizational components of memory, knowledge, and social communication (Schank & Abelson, 1995). Through narrative, humans shape their identity, ascribing meaning to oneself and to the world (McAdams, 1985, 1993; Polkinghorne, 1988).

As narratives have become increasingly accepted as central to human existence, the diverse and interdisciplinary field of narrative research has gained popularity (Spector-Mersel, 2010). Narrative researchers reject the positivist paradigm, instead operating within an interpretive-qualitative paradigm, which assumes a subjective and multifaceted social reality rather than a single objective reality (Spector-Mersel, 2010). Although life experience serves as the basis for narratives, storytelling is a creative process that provides a subjective construction of reality. In a research context, storytelling is heavily influenced by the researcher's perspective and the course of interaction between the researcher and the research participant (Rabinow & Sullivan, 1979). The storytelling process is shaped not only by the immediate context in which the story is told, but also by the larger culture and social structure in which the storyteller lives

(Plummer, 1983). Thus, narratives provide a rich representation of the complex interplay between lived experience and storyteller interpretation, as influenced by cultural and structural forces.

The rich representations of human existence that narratives provide can reflect distinct ecological levels, including the cultural, community, and individual levels. Dominant cultural narratives provide stereotypical descriptions of a particular group (e.g., dangerously unpredictable schizophrenics); community narratives are collective stories that community members share with each other (e.g., the story of the communities' founding); personal narratives are stories individuals tell about themselves (Harper et al., 2004; Mankowski & Rappaport, 2000). Life history narratives typically operate at the individual level but can also describe the history of a town, organization or other community entity. Community life histories can provide important contextual information when considered alongside the life histories of individuals who are part of the described community, thus providing insight into the reciprocal relations between community and individual.

Narratives as a Research Methodology

Life history narratives possess several strengths that make them an attractive methodological choice for researchers interested in studying complex life challenges such as mental health problems, parenting, obesity, addiction, and delinquency. Life history narratives provide a contextualized and holistic understanding of current life circumstances by tracing the history of harmful and beneficial life events (i.e., problems and solutions) that led to current circumstances. Narratives enable understanding of the dual influence of macro and micro historical events (i.e., societal- and individual-level events) on the course of an individual's life. By documenting individual accounts of the ongoing interactions between environmental circumstances and individual behavior, life history narratives explain how people came to understand themselves and their environment. This personal understanding is embedded in culture, language, gender, race, and ethnicity (Plummer, 1983).

Narrative research is also attractive from critical theory, feminist, and empowerment perspectives because narratives can provide marginalized populations with the ability to contribute to a body of knowledge about their strengths and challenges based on their own interpretations of their lives (Rappaport, 1995; Sosulski, Buchanan, & Donnell, 2010; Spector-Mersel, 2010). By examination of several narratives, where different characters struggle with a similar challenge, new insights about how to overcome the shared challenge can emerge. Thus, the analysis of several narratives focusing on a particular challenge can be an effective means of developing insight into how people can successfully overcome the challenge of interest.

Integrating Journalism and Ethnographic Research

Incorporating the use of journalism into ethnographic research raises expectations because researchers are good ethnographers and good journalists. Fortunately, expectations for the two traditions are complementary and overlap substantially. Journalism and ethnography both require rigorous honesty and penetrating analysis. Interviews, observation, attention to detail, rapport, and trust are essential to quality data collection in both disciplines.

Journalism provides ethnographic researchers with a writing style designed to produce informative and compelling narratives. Numerous textbooks and classes teach people to write journalistic feature stories, which are a specific type of journalism designed for narrative. My own training in writing journalistic feature stories consists of one undergraduate course in a school of journalism, along with exposure to the enterprise while working as a photojournalist. Once researchers become adept at using a journalistic writing style, producing it for research purposes is simply a matter of writing up the results using that style. In some studies, it may also be useful to include additional data that is not written in a journalistic style, specifically for research purposes and an academic audience.

Researchers can apply several principles of journalistic feature writing to enhance life history narratives. Journalism provides guidance on the construction of compelling lead sentences that draw the reader into the story and endings that provide the reader with closure. Frequent use of quotes is a common element of journalism that allows informants to speak for themselves in their own voice. Although a thorough explanation of journalistic writing is beyond the scope of this paper, some key points include an emphasis on the use of short sentences, short paragraphs, visual description, and flow (i.e., good use of transitions). Further, avoidance of jargon and wordiness is critical. It is important to note that the use of journalistic style is not formulaic and depends heavily on the writer's judgment.

One of the most important contributions of a journalistic style to the construction of compelling narratives is the use of narrative arc in storytelling (Friedlander & Lee, 2004). Narrative arc is a classic story structure that focuses the audience on the main character's central problems and his or her successes and failures in addressing the central problem. In this sense, use of narrative arc helps to ensure a narrative has practical value, providing the audience with a template for solving similar problems (i.e., the moral of the story; Berkow, 2001). At the beginning of a story with narrative arc, the main character is briefly established and then presented with a problem or series of obstacles that s/he strives to overcome throughout most of the story. Narratives from this study focused on mental health problems, with life experiences that enhanced coping and promoted recovery operating as the solutions. Near the end of a dramatic story with narrative arc, the main character resolves the central problem in a climactic event and the story ends. Contrived and simplistic endings are not necessary for the narrative to be compelling, however. The narratives from this study lack a climactic event where the central problem is resolved. Instead, the narratives reflect the reality that each main character has made progress in addressing his or her mental health problems, but challenges remain and there is hope for the future.

Visual Storytelling

The traditions of journalism can be guided not only by the development of narratives but also by the use of still photography and video to tell the stories of informants. These visual methods provide contextualized information about the CRO and the informants' lives that words cannot express. Consideration of the protagonist's physical presence is widely regarded as a critical component of a thorough life history narrative (Dollard, 1935; Polkinghorne, 1995). Images precisely communicate important non-verbal information such as how people present themselves to others, providing viewers with an opportunity to make judgments about the consequences of different self-presentations. Photography and film also provide detailed visual information about the activities of the CRO and the environmental context. Physical space has a profound influence on behavior (Whyte, 1980), and is essential in understanding person–environment interaction. Relevant contextual information, such as the built environment and its décor, is best communicated with images. Furthermore, photography can capture the emotions and expressions of informants in ways unparalleled by the written word. Video precisely documents the interpersonal dynamics of groups as they play out in real time. The intonations, rhythm, and pitch of spoken words maintain a vividness and subtlety that the written word cannot match. Although supplemental to the core information in written narratives, photography and video fully engage the senses and provide a complete understanding of an informant's life.

Study Setting: The P.S. Club

The P.S. Club in Wellington, Kansas, was the organizational setting in which I studied individual change processes, which occurred in 2005. I selected the P.S. Club because it was a stable CRO with relatively typically organizational pursuits and because of its proximity to my home. The Wichita State University Internal Review Board approved the study. Since 1993, the P.S. Club has been operating as an independent organization in Wellington, Kansas, a small town (pop. 8,674) 35 miles south of Wichita. In 2005, the Club had 27 active members and the equivalent of 1.75 full-time paid staff spread across four people. Although the P.S. Club is in Wellington, it serves all of Sumner County (pop. 25,256), providing transportation to and from the club to anyone in this area. The Sumner County Mental Health Center, which also provides services exclusively to the residents of Sumner County, estimated in 2005 that there were approximately 260 persons with severe and persistent mental health problems in the county, of which they served approximately 100. Based on these numbers, it is estimated that at the time of data collection, the P.S. Club had some contact with approximately 25% of those people in Sumner County who had a severe mental health problems and were receiving treatment from the public mental health system.

The P.S. Club had an annual budget of $32,822 for the 2005 fiscal year, with funds coming from the Kansas Social and Rehabilitation Services, Division of Mental Health. Like other CROs receiving state funding in Kansas, the P.S. Club maintains a drop-in center with activities that foster mutual support and provide leadership opportunities for members. In 2005, the Club was open from 10 am to 4 pm, Monday through Friday. During this time, members had potluck meals, card games, business meetings, and pool games on a regular basis. Additional organizational pursuits included making presentations in the community to increase public awareness about mental health problems and operating a warm line for people to call when they wanted to talk to a peer counselor. A warm line is similar to a mental health hotline, except it is not intended for use during emergencies. There are several different ways members can get involved, such as organizing CRO activities, becoming a board member or hired staff, or helping in maintaining the facility. Participants from the P.S. Club do not represent the entire population of people who participate in CROs in Kansas or nationally, but the P.S. Club has relatively typical organizational pursuits for a CRO. Despite some inevitable organizational differences, transferring findings to other settings is still possible because readers can use the detailed information about the P.S. Club to help make judgments about how well the findings from this study can inform different settings.

Study Sample

A theoretical approach (Strauss & Corbin, 1998) guided the sampling of P.S. Club members for the development of life histories. The theoretical approach emphasized the selection of informants based on the perspective and information they brought to the study and to the exploration of theory. I selected informants primarily from among those people who were deeply involved in the P.S. Club. The CRO had a core group of 5–10 regular attendees and it was these members, rather than those who sporadically attended, who were the primary focus of this research. Because this study focused on understanding the extent to which CRO involvement can impact the lives of participants, four of the seven informants selected were people deeply involved in the organization – Mary, Carl, Nick, and Kevin. The perspectives of people who are less involved in the organization are also important in understanding CROs. Therefore, one new member (Laura) and one member who had recently disengaged from the organization (Joe) were interviewed. Additionally, I included one individual who "graduated" from a different CRO and now provides technical assistance to the P.S. Club (Sue). Sue provided a perspective that current P.S. Club members cannot provide: that of someone who had used a CRO for self-improvement and then moved on to accomplish other life goals.

Together, these seven informants provided as much theoretical variation as could be attained within this relatively small CRO. The study was limited to one CRO because of resource limitations. Substantial resources had to be invested in a single CRO in order to obtain the depth and breadth of knowledge necessary to understand personal transformations, which are a complex and private matter. Understanding personal transformations requires the researcher to develop close relationships with each informant. Intensive study of a few informants can effectively serve as a basis for theory building because it allows the researcher to further conceptual thinking rather than simply test current hypotheses. Theorists who have effectively used this strategy include Piaget (1952), Erikson (1950), and Borkman (1999).

Participant Observation

Participant observation combined participation in the lives of the CRO members with maintenance of a professional distance that allowed adequate observation and recording of data. Estroff (1981, p. 20) summarized well the dilemma of using participant observation methods to understand people with mental health problems:

> The anthropological field worker customarily attempts to learn and to reach understanding through asking, doing, watching, testing, and experiencing for herself the same activities, rituals, rules, and meanings as the subjects. Our subjects become the experts, the instructors, and we become the students (Blumer 1969; Maretzki 1973). But if we are studying persons who are crazy (i.e., actively psychotic or living the crazy life), we are restricted in reaching optimal levels of experience and participation in the subjects' world if we are to remain sane.

Although this is a barrier to participant observation, the method remains nonetheless critical in providing a rich understanding of the lives of the informants. Furthermore, psychiatric diagnoses are not the primary focus of the P.S. Club. Although the Club is for people with mental health problems, its activities emphasize recreation and friendship, resembling that of any socially focused organization.

I observed participants at the P.S. Club 32 times over an 18-month period. Observation sessions typically lasted between 3 and 4 h. During my first visit to the P.S. Club, I administered an organizational health questionnaire and an organizational activity questionnaire (see Appendices A and B). Although everyone responded positively to the questionnaire, I was labeled as a researcher evaluating the organization.

After administering the questionnaire, I began working with P.S. Club members on photovoice project. Photovoice is a participatory action research methodology where community members use cameras to generate and interpret their own data. Originally developed by Caroline Wang and colleagues, the process can empower participants by enabling a greater degree of participant control over what data are collected and how they are interpreted (Wang & Burris, 1997; Wang & Redwood-Jones, 2001). The goal of the photovoice project was to illustrate what goes on at the P.S. Club and how people benefit from the experience.

I implemented the project in collaboration with Sue, a fellow employee at the Center for Community Support & Research. Sue was the primary technical assistance provider to the P.S. Club, a person with mental health problems, and a person whose story is told in this study. Implementing photovoice consisted of handing out cameras, showing people how to use them, providing some tips on how to take good pictures, and discussing as a group what pictures people might want to take.

One-on-one interviews with the photographers and those photographed were then used to interpret the photos. The project required six weekly visits to the P.S. Club, as cameras were handed out three times and data interpreted three times. For the latter half of the project, Sue's help became unnecessary and I started going to the P.S. Club by myself.

The photovoice project provided important insight into the P.S. Club and its members (Brown, Collins, Shepherd, Wituk, & Meissen, 2004). The implementation process was important in developing rapport with P.S. Club members. Everyone enjoyed the free cameras, film, pictures, and candy that came with the experience. The experience helped to form a trusting relationship between myself and the leadership of the organization. My initial label as an evaluation researcher led to some social desirability bias on the part of the P.S. Club's leadership, who wanted to promote a positive evaluation of the organization. However, working with the organization on a project enjoyed by all, trust emerged as it became clear that my intentions were to help the organization. My label as evaluation researcher dissipated and the motivation to provide a socially desirable presentation relaxed.

Following the implementation of photovoice, I started simply showing up, playing games, and socializing with the P.S. Club members. Over time, as relationships developed with P.S. Club members, I started asking to attend and began being invited to join in activities outside of the P.S. Club. Observations made outside the context of the P.S. Club allowed for placement of the CRO participation experience into the broader context of each person's life. With Kevin, I went to a concert and two festivals organized by Caldwell, KS, the small town in which he lived. With Carl and Mary, I went to two parades and a fair. With Joe I went out to eat, to shop at Dollar General, and to a museum where he volunteers.

Only one person was interested in showing me their home. Of all the interviewees, Sue was the only person who chose her home as the preferred place to do interviews. Carl and Mary were willing, but only because that is where I wanted to interview them. Nick and Joe both said their place was too messy. Kevin was reluctant, not wanting to show me the inside at first, and wanted us do interviews so the neighbor's nicer house was visible in the background. Laura preferred the idea of doing interviews at the P.S. Club. This trend, which interfered with the attainment of good observational data outside of the CRO, may partially be due to the low incomes of the group and modest-to-substandard housing conditions of most of P.S. Club members. As someone with a full-time job requiring higher education, Sue stood as an exception to this rule as well.

As a participant observer, I socialized and participated in P.S. Club activities in much the same way other members did. However, I was working on a photo and video documentary of the P.S. Club during my visits, and my use of cameras distinguished me from others. My participant observation was not traditional in the sense that I did not regularly write notes while in the field. Instead, I used the video camera as a note-taking device. Immediately after returning from a participant observation experience, I would review my pictures and video footage. From these data and my own memory of the experience, I would write down relevant incidences and reflections on what occurred during my observation. I chose this strategy primarily because taking notes while trying to take pictures and capture video was overly burdensome.

As time progressed, my rapport with P.S. Club members became quite strong. However, I was never viewed as regular member of the Club. I always maintained the special status of graduate student, photographer, and employee of the Center for Community Support & Research, which provided technical assistance to CROs across Kansas. There were also socioeconomic differences between myself and most P.S. Club members. Although these class differences did not pose a major barrier, they were clearly present. Just as I was struck by the simplicity of their potluck, I am sure P.S. Club members found some of my own behavior curious. Nevertheless, many members came to view me as a regular attendee, and began to wonder what had happened if I was not present for a week or more. P.S. Club members also adjusted to the presence of cameras and increasingly ignored my use of them. By the end of the study, I had developed a strong relationship with all regular attendees, especially those whose life history narratives I wrote. In fact, after data collection was complete and it was clear I was soon going to move away, I received an honorary plaque from the P.S. Club for my service to their organization.

Minimally Structured Interviews

A series of in-depth, minimally structured interviews (MSIs) served as the primary data source in the development of life histories. During the interviews, I worked to obtain a developmental understanding of where people spent their time and how that has changed over the years. I wanted to understand the challenges each person faced, how those challenges have influenced development, and what each has done to overcome those challenges. I strove for understanding of the de-integrating and re-integrating experiences over the life course. Additionally, identity theory (Burke, Owens, Serpe, & Thoits, 2003; Stryker, 1980; Stryker & Burke, 2000) guided the interviews into some specific topics of interest including that of social networks, social roles, skill development, and individual identity.

I conducted the interviews in an iterative fashion, gathering more information as analysis deemed necessary. Typically, I interviewed informants for two or three 60-min sessions. Interviewing ceased when saturation had been reached (i.e., new information was not being uncovered) and life histories could be written. Informants were reimbursed at the rate of $15 per 60-min interview session.

I used minimal structure during interviews to allow informants to tell their stories in their own words and according to their own understanding of the experience, rather than guided by my own preconceived notions. Although the interviews varied significantly from person to person, I developed a starting point interview protocol guided by the role framework to provide the interviews with some structure. I divided this protocol into four segments: (a) community involvement, (b) social networks, (c) personal background, and (d) identity, skills, and goals.

The community involvement segment examined the routines of each informant and how each had evolved over time, with a particular emphasis on CRO involvement. The social networks segment examined the development of personal relationships over time and the consequences of each relationship for each informant. The personal background segment provided a general and broad understanding of the history and culture of the informant, including education, upbringing, religious background, employment, and psychiatric history. In the identity, skills, and goals interview segment I attempted to understand the interrelationships between individual identity, role relationships, and skill development. Information on goals, obstacles, and problem solving was also a focus of this interview segment.

Although I created this framework to guide entry into the study, as the interviews progressed, it became increasingly obsolete. I abandoned many of the questions partway through the study because they did not elicit information helpful in telling the life histories of each informant. While early interviews used a more semi-structured format, later interviews were more unstructured. The less structured format simply proved to be more efficient and effective in eliciting the information necessary to write thorough life histories.

During interviews, I frequently used follow-up questions, which served two basic purposes. One was to elicit more detail. These questions were typically quite simple, such as, "Could you explain further?" "Could you give me an example" and *"Really?"*. The other common follow-up was intended to reflect back my own understanding of what the interviewee said, making sure we maintained a shared understanding.

Interviews took place after I completed most of the participant observation. The rapport that developed during participant observation allowed me to ask several uncomfortable questions frankly and receive honest answers during interviews. Furthermore, the rich but frequently happenstance personal information obtained during participant observation allowed me to ask more poignant questions. The interviews provided opportunities to organize much of the participant observation data into more coherent and chronological life histories.

It is important to note that participant observation and minimally structured interviews collect two different types of stories (Spector-Mersel, 2010). During participant observation, researchers collect stories that narrators produce in naturalistic settings for audiences other than the researcher. In contrast, during minimally structured interviews, research participants produce stories for the researcher through interactions with the researcher. Although researcher presence influences storytelling in both settings, the influence is substantially more prominent during interviews because storytelling depends on the purpose of the study and the interview questions generated by the researcher.

Life History Construction

The construction of life history narratives served as an analytic strategy for organizing and synthesizing the enormous amount of data collected during fieldwork into a coherent developmental account of the life under study. The minimally structured interviews were both a critical source of information for narrative construction and as a medium for communicating the insider's perspective. Quotes allowed informants to speak for themselves, thereby enabling the individual life histories to provide an emic or insider's perspective on how CROs can be beneficial. Although I attempted to convey an emic perspective with the narratives, my etic perspective heavily influenced narrative construction. I decided which quotes to present and I organized those quotes in a manner consistent with my understanding of the life history described by informants. To help keep the narratives consistent with an insider's perspective, I engaged in participant observation, which helped me understand CRO participation from an emic perspective. The blend of emic and etic perspectives in life history narratives is similar to the writings of traditional ethnographic material, where the authors blend data from the field with their own understanding of the situation.

Additionally shaping the narrative content was my interest in understanding how the mental health and well-being of informants changed over time, along with how their CRO involvement influenced their health and well-being. Further, I paid attention to life experiences relating to constructs within the role framework. However, I remained committed to understanding the insider perspective and communicating life experiences deemed important by the informant, just as my interview questions followed the informant's lead.

Life history construction began with a careful review of all field notes and interview transcripts pertaining to a particular informant. Facilitating this process was the coding, by name, of all field notes and interview transcripts that referenced a particular informant, using QSR International's qualitative data analysis software package NUD*IST 6 (2002). During review of the informant-specific text, I noted all information I deemed pertinent to understanding an individual's life history. More specifically, I noted all life experiences relating to mental health problems, personal challenges, community involvement, personal relationship developments, individual strengths, skill development, personal goals, identity, recovery progress, and changing daily routines. I also noted all poignant and insightful quotes describing the life experiences previously identified as relevant. All of these notes combined to make a list of data relevant to the life story.

Next, I organized all notes chronologically to create detailed accounts of each informant's life. Wherever possible, I triangulated observational and interview data to improve the accuracy of the detailed chronological timelines. During the process of organizing each life history, I revealed gaps in my own understanding of each informant. To address this problem, I wrote follow-up questions for informants and used brief phone conversations or asides during participant observation to fill in gaps in understanding. Narrative construction at this stage was not simply a matter of information organization, however. I also noticed connections between disparate events and gained insight into the causes and consequences of different life events. Although these connections and insights were initially tentative, I was able to verify them in subsequent conversations.

Constructing a detailed life history timeline facilitated the identification of a central plot that drove each informant's life. The plot connected various life events and happenings, providing an explanation of how the events lead to a particular outcome (Polkinghorne, 1995). In the study, the particular outcome of interest was the mental health and community integration of each informant during data collection. Recursive movement between the data and the emerging story outline enables plot identification and refinement. Data from the field was a chaotic mix of relevant and irrelevant life events. Development of a plot helped the narrative analysis focus on life events that influenced mental health and community integration (Polkinghorne, 1995). As such plot identification was critical from both a storytelling and an analytic perspective, it made the story more compelling and focused on consequential life events.

The focus provided by plot refinement facilitated the transition from detailed life history timeline to the construction of a detailed narrative outline. To aid narrative organization, I also used a problem-and-solution structure that is similar to the narrative arc used in journalistic feature writing and other types of stories. This problem-and-solution structure led me to present negative experiences and personal challenges (i.e., the problems) early in each narrative. Later in the narratives were the solutions – the positive experiences, individual strengths, and skill development. It is important to note that I did not rigidly enforce the use of a problem and solution story sequence. Rather, I used the story structure when it was consistent with the data and could help organize it in a manner that promoted a coherent and accurate account of the informants' life histories. Generally, it was fitting because informants developed mental health problems earlier in life and were in the process of recovery when I met them. Use of a problem and solution structure promoted an understanding of how the role relationships and daily routines maintained when life was worsening differed from the role relationships and daily routines maintained when life was improving. As further described in the results, understanding how role relationships and life circumstances relate to one another proved fundamental to drawing conclusions about how CRO roles and relationships influenced behavior and well-being.

In order to provide the life history narratives with rich contextual background, I also created narratives describing the P.S. Club and the mental health system in Wellington. These narratives illustrate how CROs fit into the larger mental health system. Furthermore, the culture of the P.S. Club and the larger context of the mental health system have a profound influence on the behavior of informants. Such contextual information is essential to understanding the conditions that promote personal transformation within informants.

Analysis of Narratives

For theory development to occur, researchers must consider the data from an etic or outsider's perspective. As such, each individual life history has an individual theoretical analysis presented in Chap. 6. Here, I made connections between the informant's experiences and the conceptual framework in an effort to understand how the lives of informants can and cannot be understood and described by the role framework.

When I found inconsistencies, I explored the use of alternative theoretical explanations. This stage of analysis is akin to ethnographic interpretation (LeCompte & Schensul, 1999), where the insider's understanding is connected to the literature and brought to bear on the primary research question of how people benefit from CROs.

Life history narratives were also analyzed to identify recurring themes that appear across cases. As organized summaries of important life events and personal development, the condensed nature of the narratives facilitated the discovery of empirically grounded patterns and themes (LeCompte & Schensul, 1999). Identified patterns and themes provide insight into how change processes described by the role framework play out in real life. Contextual information in the narratives enables understanding of why different people experience difference change processes. Understanding these differences is critical to understanding what needs to occur and what needs to be avoided for CRO participation experiences to promote recovery. The summary cross-case analysis of narratives at the end of Chap. 6 also provides insight into how the narratives validate and contradict the role framework.

Sharing Narratives

The final step in the narrative construction process was the sharing of narratives and subsequent theoretical analyses with each informant. I did this primarily to ensure accuracy of the narratives. It also provided informants with an opportunity to remove elements of the narrative they were not comfortable sharing with others. Although I gave everyone the opportunity to censor any aspect of his or her story s/he was uncomfortable with, only one informant was inclined to do so. Although the excluded information did illustrate important concepts, these concepts remain illustrated by several other examples. The information omission did not contradict any conclusions made in this study. Separate consent forms were used to obtain permission to share pictures and life histories of informants with the general public. However, because I altered some of the theoretical analyses of life histories after obtaining consent, I use pseudonyms in this book.

Conclusion

Life histories tell the individual stories of informants, examining the joys, pains, triumphs, and difficulties of each person's life. The underlying goal of narrative construction was to provide insight into how CRO participation altered the lives of informants. Such explanations lay the groundwork for exploring the degree of congruency between data and theory. Chapter 5 presents the life history narratives developed for this study and Chap. 6 analyzes those narratives, providing insight into how the theoretical framework can and cannot account for the lived experience of CRO participants.

Chapter 5
Life History Narratives from the P.S. Club

Abstract This chapter presents the colorful narratives of seven participants in a consumer-run organization (CRO), called the P.S. Club. The narratives illustrate how the lives of participants developed over time and how their involvement in the P.S. Club changed their life course. The extensive use of quotes helps to provide an insiders' understanding of the challenges people with mental health problems face and the nature of CRO participation. Documentary photography helps bring each narrative to life, providing informative visual information that cannot be communicated through words. To enhance the contextual description, the chapter also provides a narrative describing life inside the local mental health system and a narrative specifically exploring the P.S. Club as an organization.

Life Inside Wellington's Mental Health System

West Mineral, Kansas, is home to the world's largest electric shovel. Garden City, Kansas, is home to the largest cow hairball. Every town has its claim to fame, but only Wellington is the wheat capital of the world (Fig. 5.1).

While these claims may provide residents with a sense of pride and identity, their reasons for staying run much deeper. Trains, airplanes, and wheat provide many Wellington residents with jobs. Churches and high school sports provide a social fabric, weaving the town together. Both large enough for a variety of activities and small enough for people to know each other, many residents consider Wellington to be the perfect size.

Unnoticed by the average resident, however, are the mental health services available in Wellington. Having a psychiatric diagnosis provides a whole new perspective on what Wellington has to offer.

Mary is one resident all too familiar with this perspective (Fig. 5.2). Mary has been diagnosed with schizoaffective disorder, bipolar type, meaning that she experiences the symptoms of schizophrenia, along with major depressive and manic episodes. Anxiety, depression, paranoia, and hallucinations are all horribly familiar.

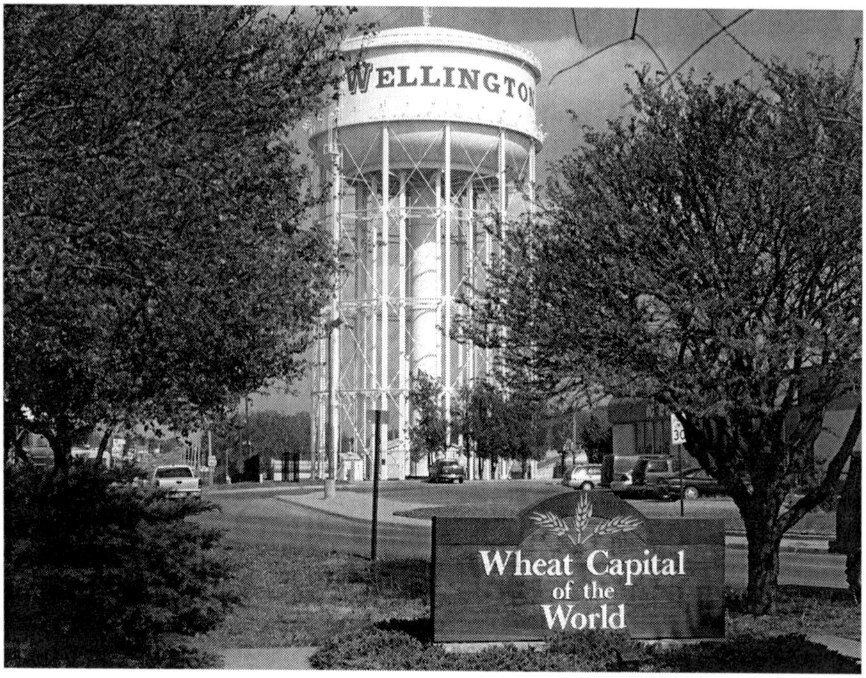

Fig. 5.1 The P.S. Club is located in the small town of Wellington, Kansas (pop. 8421)

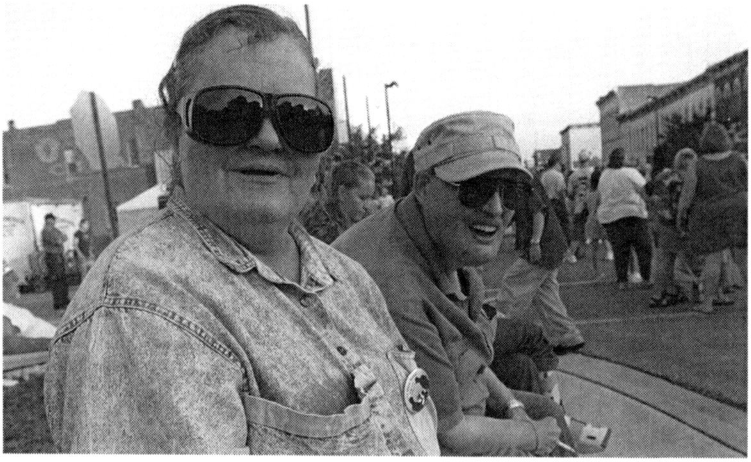

Fig. 5.2 Mary and Carl are good friends who go many places together. Pictured here, they enjoy the Wellington Parade together

Fortunately, Mary is relatively well cared for through a wide variety of mental health services. Employing more than 70 people and serving more than 2,000 clients, the mental health system stands as a major industry in Wellington.

Serving as the fulcrum of this system is the Sumner Mental Health Center. A product of deinstitutionalization, the center provides mental health services to adults and children with the goal of helping people live healthy lives in the community, rather than isolated in psychiatric hospitals. The mental health center has 11 licensed therapists, who provide therapy to both children and adults. Mary sees her therapist about every other week, where they "just talk about stuff and everything," says Mary.

In addition, there is one part-time psychiatrist and one Advanced Registered Nurse Practitioner (ARNP), who provide medication for both mental and physical health problems. They help Mary strike a balance between all of her different medications and their side effects.

In addition to therapy and medication management, the Sumner Mental Health Center provides Mary with case management and attendant care. Mary's case manager helps with the coordination of care. She sees Mary about twice a month, working with her to plan a budget, set daily living goals, and manage symptoms.

While case managers focus on planning, attendant care workers focus on the implementation of these plans. Further differentiating these two positions is level of education. Attendant care workers must have a high school diploma while case managers need a bachelor's degree. Mary's attendant care worker visits 4 days a week for 2 h a day, helping her around the house and taking her shopping and to the doctor. She also enjoys recreational activities with Mary occasionally, taking her to the lake to fish and feed the ducks.

Vocational services are one of the few resources Mary does not take advantage of. That is because she already has a job working at the P.S. Club on Mondays, Thursdays, and Fridays. The P.S. Club is a nonprofit operated by people with mental health problems. Through grants and contract work, the club hosts recreational activities, provides peer support, and makes presentations in the community about mental health problems. Mary works as a shift manager, answering the phone and cleaning up the building after a day of activity (Fig. 5.3). Along with employment, the P.S. Club serves as her primary source of social support. When she is not working there, she goes to the club simply to enjoy a game of pool or chat with her friends.

When Mary wants to go places, she calls Futures Unlimited for a $2 van ride. Although this service sounds simple enough, most towns do not have subsidized transportation. Futures Unlimited is a developmental disability organization that provides this service through a grant from the Kansas Department of Transportation and local matching funds. "You just call them up, and they'll tell you when they can be there," says Mary.

Being on disability also impacts Mary's housing situation. Her apartment complex is subsidized by the U.S. Department of Housing and Urban Development (HUD). The apartment complex takes 30% of her monthly Social Security Income (SSI) check in return for a basic, one-bedroom dwelling. For the apartment complex

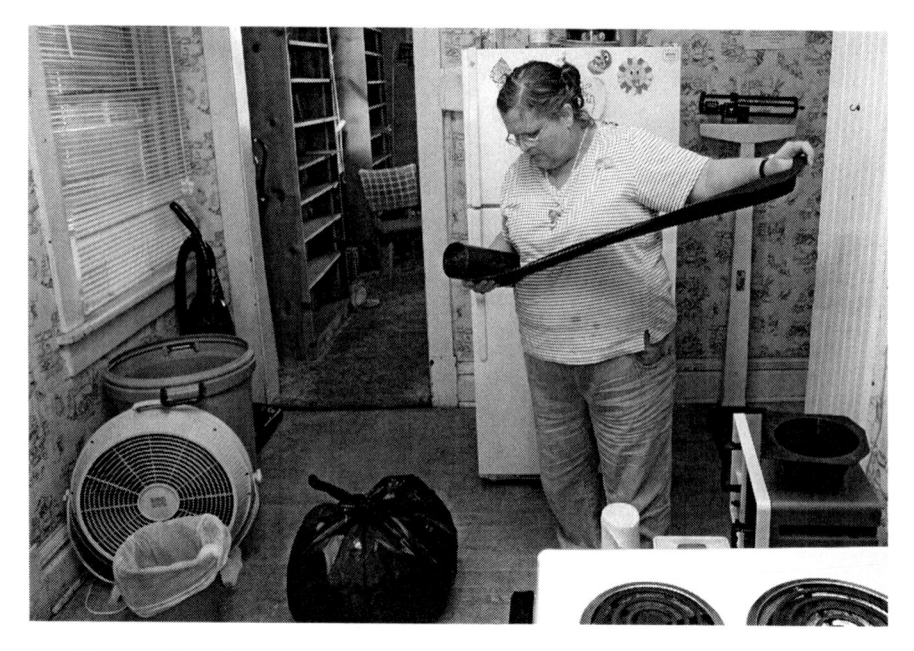

Fig. 5.3 One of Mary's chores at the P.S. Club is to take out the trash

to remain profitable, HUD covers the difference between what comes from SSI and the market value of the apartment.

Interfacing with the mental health system are the police, who frequently get involved when psychiatric symptoms overwhelm a person. Unfortunately, Mary recently went through such an experience. Her paranoia grew out control and she began to fear her friend was going to kill her with a butcher knife and burn the apartment down with cigarettes. She called the police, who took her to Sumner Regional Medical Center, the hospital in Wellington. The hospital has a psychiatric ward that primarily serves elderly people with dementia and Alzheimer's. While there her condition only worsened. When friends came to visit and bring her clothes she did not recognize them. After a few days Mary was involuntarily committed to Larned State Hospital as a last resort.

For the first 5 days at Larned, Mary did nothing but sleep. Upon awakening, Mary had absolutely no idea where she was or what happened. Unfortunately a psychotic consciousness was regained and the hospital did not provide an environment conducive to recovery. Full of harrowing screams and "a lot of different people up there with a lot of problems" according to Mary, mental hospitals frequently provide an environment that stands as the exact opposite of what someone with schizophrenia needs.

Schizophrenia can be intensely confusing. Thoughts race, time warps, imaginations run wild, and the real cannot be separated from the unreal. Paranoia from the confusion can quickly set in. Hearing other people's agony in a hospital setting can provide fodder for your own agonizing and relentless imagination.

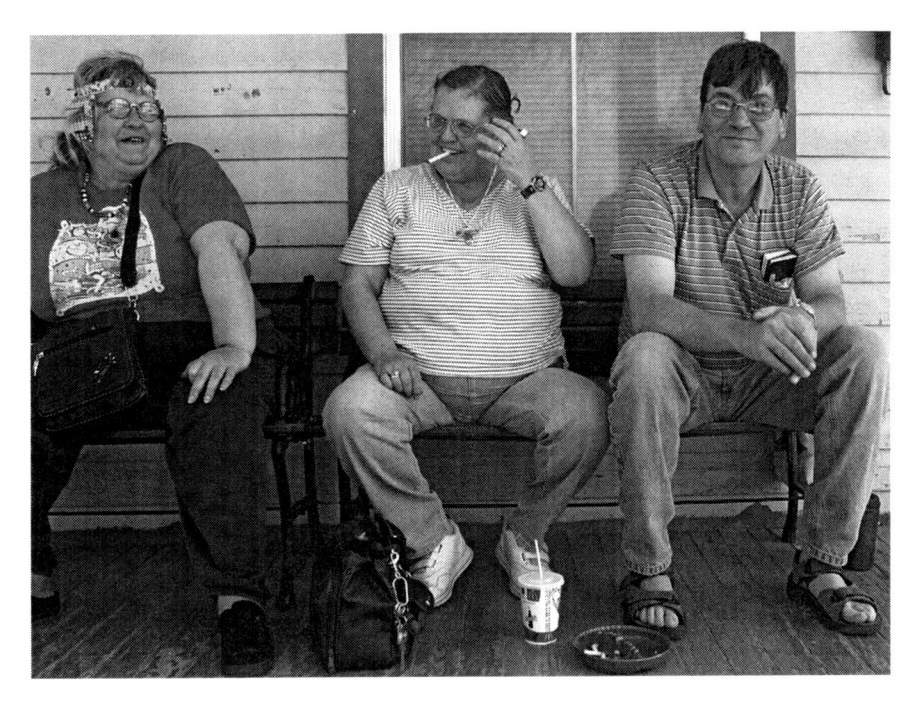

Fig. 5.4 Mary enjoys the company of her friends at the P.S. Club

Mary recalls one of her own psychotic episodes at the hospital. "I was in the bathroom beating my head on the floor. I did that for about 30 min." She adds, "It took me 2 weeks before I could even go to the cafeteria because there was so many people up there that I got too paranoid. I was hearing voices and hallucinations and the voices were controlling me."

With handcuffs on her wrists and chains around her feet, Mary was escorted by the police 173 miles from the Larned State Hospital to the Sumner County Courthouse, where it was decided she was not ready to come home. The court hearing was required by law because Mary was involuntarily committed.

Anxious to get back to a normal life in Wellington with her friends at the P.S. Club, she worked hard to meet all the self-care requirements of release and in 6 weeks she went home. "I was just glad to be able to come home and be alive. Every night I'd go to sleep thinking I was going to die and never wake up." Mary recalls.

Mary is now stable again, and while she still has many problems to overcome, she has a job, a group of friends, and clarity to her thoughts (Fig. 5.4). "Right now I feel like a brand new person since I got out of Larned and finally got my medicine straightened out and it got into my system. Man, I go to bed a 9 O'clock at night, get up every morning at 6 and I feel great," she says. "I feel better than I have in my whole life!" Compared to Larned, Wellington offers Mary pure paradise.

Facing Serious Mental Health Problems, Running a Nonprofit

Schizophrenia creates a reality that doesn't exist. "I thought all kinds of things were going on and all I was really doing was sitting there, staring at the wall," says Nick, who has been diagnosed with schizophrenia.

Confused, discombobulated, scared, a mental breakdown occurs. "It was hell. I mean, I have never been through so much hell in all my life," Mary recalls from her most recent mental breakdown. "Every night I would go to sleep I was thinking I was going to die and I'd never wake up."

The work of sorting the real from the unreal is never ending. All perceptions must be questioned, and paranoia easily sets in. Mary recalls feeling, "too paranoid and too nervous, I wouldn't get out of my apartment." Self-soothing becomes a full-time job. Cigarettes help.

Few understand what you are facing. "They just hear the name schizophrenia and they automatically think you are a bad person," recounts Nick. While the cause is unknown, schizophrenia is experienced by 1% of the population.

Major depression is another common diagnosis. Abused as a child, Carl described his experiences with major depression. He had persistent negative thoughts, such as "I'm worthless, I'm no good," he remembers.

Over time, Carl's feelings led to episodes of major depression, where life became misery. Thoughts such as "I'll never amount to anything" regularly ran though his mind. Apathy overwhelmed him. At times, it became hard to justify his misery when he didn't see any point to life. "There have been times that I tried suicide," he says.

A multitude of other disorders and subtypes exist, but schizophrenia and depression account for the majority of psychiatric diagnoses.

Social isolation frequently exacerbates mental health problems. Nick pegs stigma as one of the primary causes. "So many people out there, they have no idea what mental illness is. All they ever see is, you know, in the movies or on the news when something bad happens. And that makes them fearful and it makes it really difficult for a person with a mental illness to get out and make friends," he says.

Kevin is one man who has trouble developing close relationships. "I just stay here at the house, watching TV, watching TV," he says. With no relationships, no laughs to share, and no shoulder to cry on, the world is a cold place (Fig. 5.5).

Isolation leads people with schizophrenia to develop depression and people with depression sink further into despair. Many basic needs go unfulfilled, such as love, a sense of belonging, purpose in life, and a feeling of being needed. "Just for happiness in life, everybody needs friends," says Nick.

The P.S. Club stands as an organization trying to solve this problem. Named after the post script in letters that often say P.S. I love you, the P.S. Club is a place where people with mental health problems find acceptance and support (Fig. 5.6). Nick is the executive director. Carl is the president of the board of directors. Mary is the treasurer of the board and Kevin is a regular attendee.

The club fills an important gap in the mental health system because "people with mental illness, they want the same kinds of relationships and stuff that people that don't have a mental illness want," says Nick. "They want someone to care about, someone to be there for them."

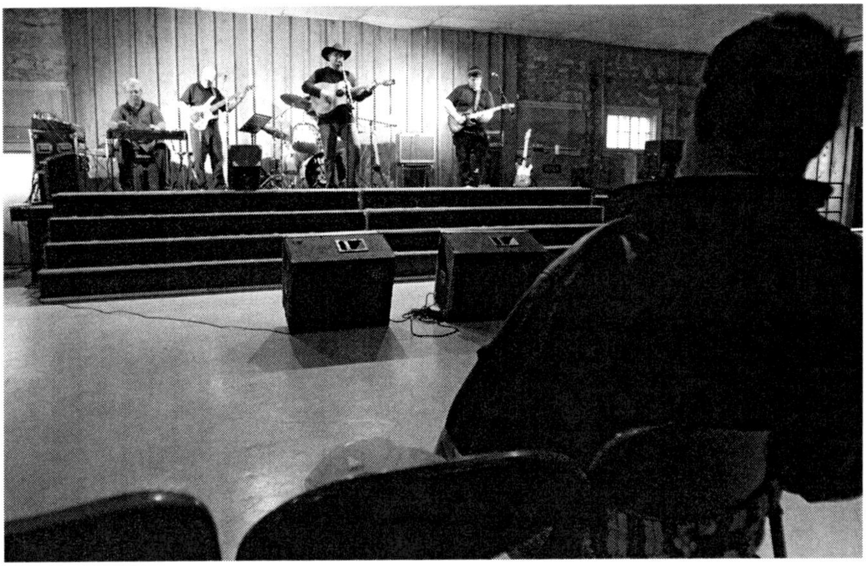

Fig. 5.5 Kevin watches Kelly Dennison perform at a free concert. Kevin was excited about the show months ahead of time. He encouraged many people to go but he ended up going by himself

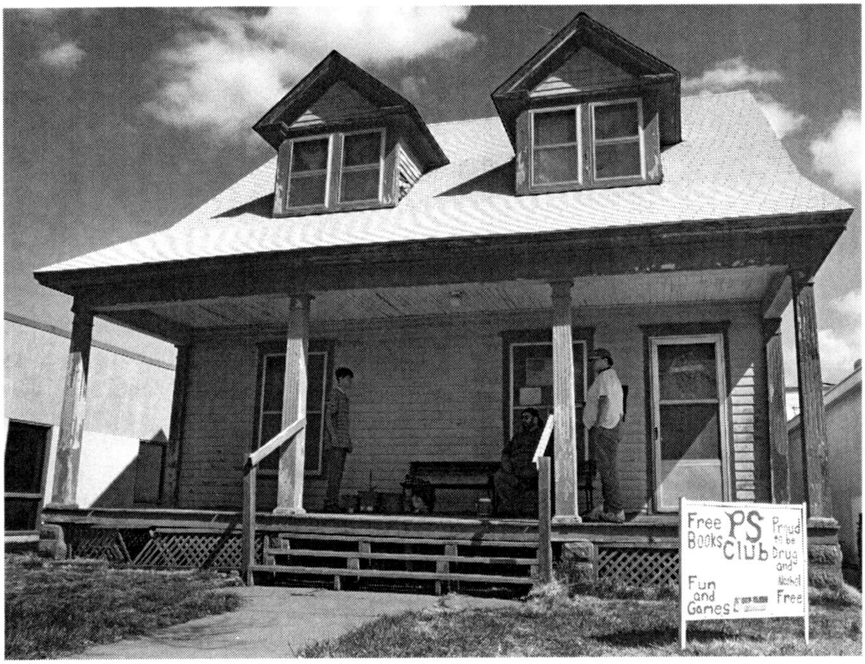

Fig. 5.6 The P.S. Club pays $300 a month to rent a house owned by the Sumner Mental Health Center

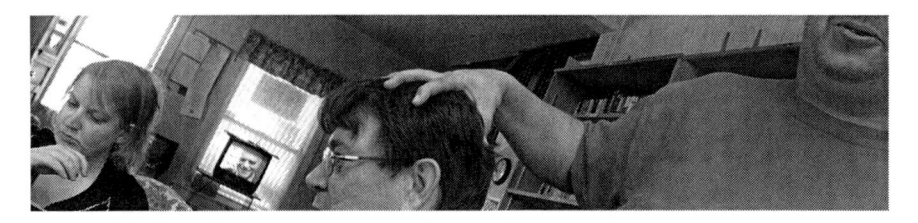

Fig. 5.7 The P.S. Club is often a place of smiles and playfulness

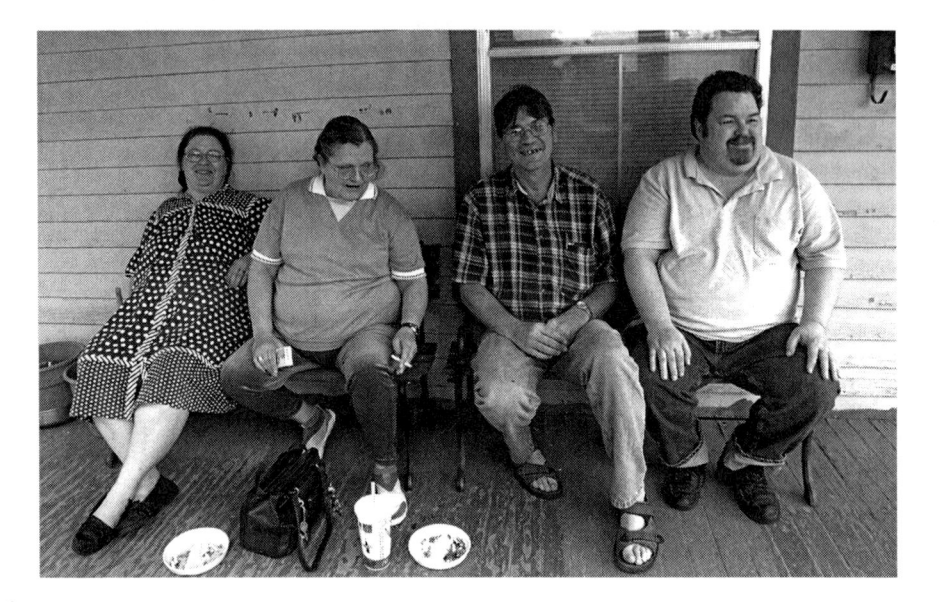

Fig. 5.8 When the weather is nice, the porch outside of the P.S. Club is a favorite hangout. It is not uncommon for members to spend the better part of the day sitting outside telling stories

The club is located in the small town of Wellington, Kansas, where people can drop-in and socialize. It provides a friendly and safe atmosphere. "I like to have fun with people, not make fun of people, because nobody has fun that way," says Carl to a newcomer at the club (Fig. 5.7).

Conversations range from somber condolences to simple memories. For example, one afternoon several members were reminiscing about the good old days. "We used to go to the drugstore down there and they'd sell Cherry Cokes," said Nick. Carl warmly replied with fondness. "Oh, that's when you could really taste the cherry." Everyone agreed in unison (Fig. 5.8).

Mutual support is a key element of the social interactions at the P.S. Club. One member who visited the club after a recent hospitalization was quickly surrounded by supportive words. "I can definitely say that I understand what you're going through because I've been through it myself," said Carl. "I'd rather see you do the things you need to do instead of get sick and have to go back."

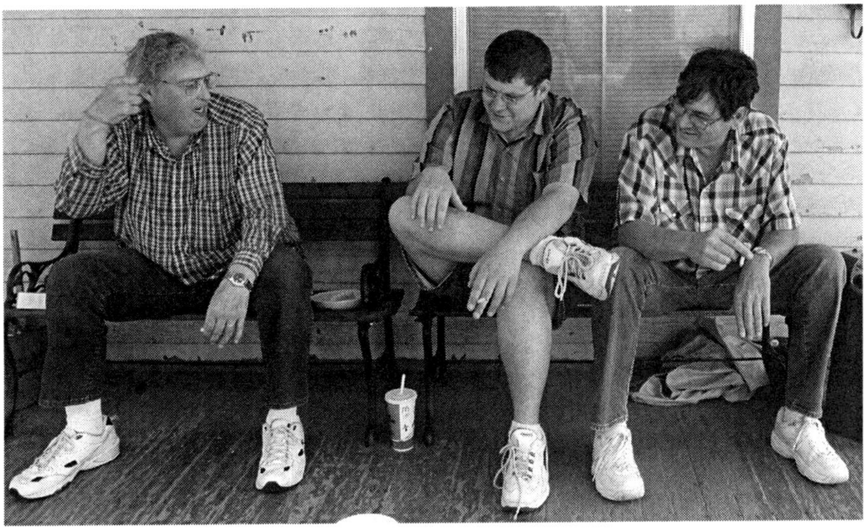

Fig. 5.9 Carl enjoys telling a funny story to fellow P.S. Club members. He honed his ability to maintain lighthearted interactions through his many visits to the club

Joking and silly stories are also part of the lighthearted atmosphere (Fig. 5.9). Nick remembers one joke with John fondly. "[John] always talked about wanting a good looking woman. I said a new one joined the club here the other day. He goes, 'Oh Wow, where is she at?' Then [Brian, a large hairy man] come out off the back porch in that dress and started chasing him around," he recalls with a hearty laugh. "[John] turned about 14 different colors of red."

Even singing breaks out occasionally, as one member volunteered the following tune:

> I went to the church just the other night.
> There I saw Jesus he was out of sight.
> I said to Jesus, "Hey JC, Oh won't you pray for me?
> Won't you Won't you Won't you pray for me?"

The conversations help people develop lasting relationships. "I've told [Nick] things that I wouldn't tell anybody else or he has told me things that he wouldn't tell anybody else," says Carl. "That's a good feeling to be able to talk to somebody like that, and know that they trust you also."

The support people receive buffers stress and improves daily coping. "It's easier to cope when you're not stressed really bad and when you've got other people to socialize with," says Nick. "A lot of that will relieve a part of your stress, you know, just getting with other people and playing games and stuff and not worrying about whatever problems you think you might have at the time" (Fig. 5.10).

When members aren't talking, they are playing games such as pool, cards, or board games (Figs. 5.11–5.14). These games provide a medium for more lighthearted joking. During a game of "Sorry," Katie took some of Carl's pieces and joked, "Hahaha, I'm a mean sucker aren't I?" But Carl knew he was going to have his

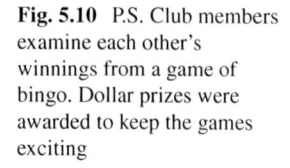

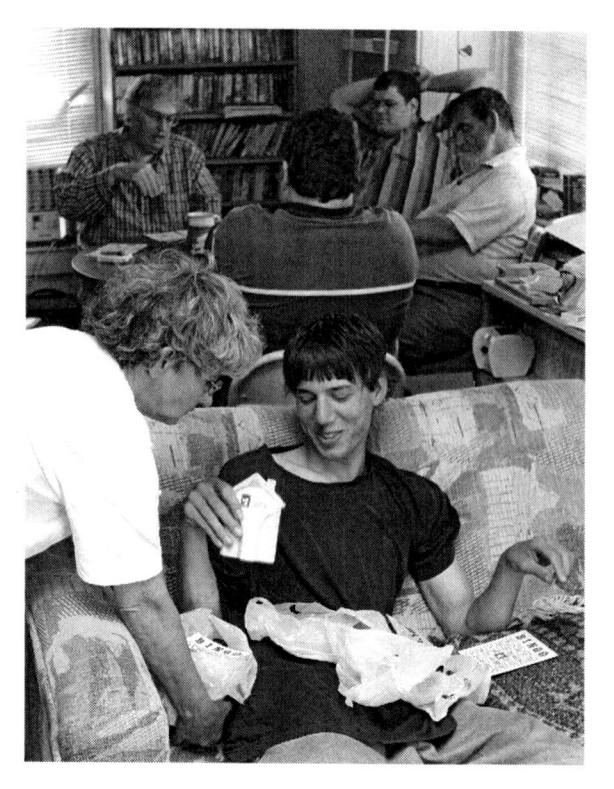

Fig. 5.10 P.S. Club members examine each other's winnings from a game of bingo. Dollar prizes were awarded to keep the games exciting

revenge after peaking at the card he was about to draw. "So am I, So am I!" he said with enthusiasm. Confused, Katie replied, "Ok, if you say so." But then she quickly realized the meaning of his words when he knocked her pieces back to home, playfully shouting, "Hey! You're mean!" To which everyone was amused.

Cookouts and movie days are also regularly scheduled. The recreational activities improve quality of life. "Just getting up here and playing cards and games and stuff with people- I really enjoy that and shooting pool on Fridays. It's just kind of a big stress relief for me," says Nick. Kevin agrees. "It seems like just every time I go there I have a good time," he says.

The recreational activities serve as a medium for the development of lasting friendships. In turn, the friendships can serve as a powerful antidepressant. Carl attributes a large part of his recovery from depression to his socializing at the club (Fig. 5.15). "I think a lot of it has to do with me just coming to the clubhouse. Having somebody to talk to," he says.

What makes the P.S. Club truly unique is that it is operated entirely by people with mental health problems. These types of organizations are a new and growing development within the mental health system and there are now 21 such nonprofits in Kansas today. The P.S. Club opened its doors in 1993, when Nick wrote a grant to the Kansas Department of Social and Rehabilitation Services.

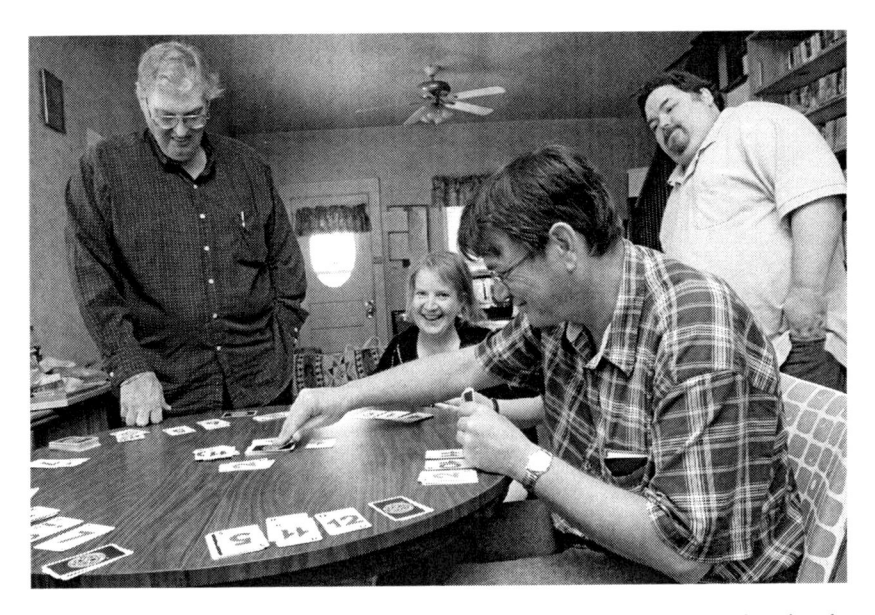

Fig. 5.11 Cards are one of the most popular activities at the P.S. Club. Lighthearted teasing about the luck and misfortunes of other players is common

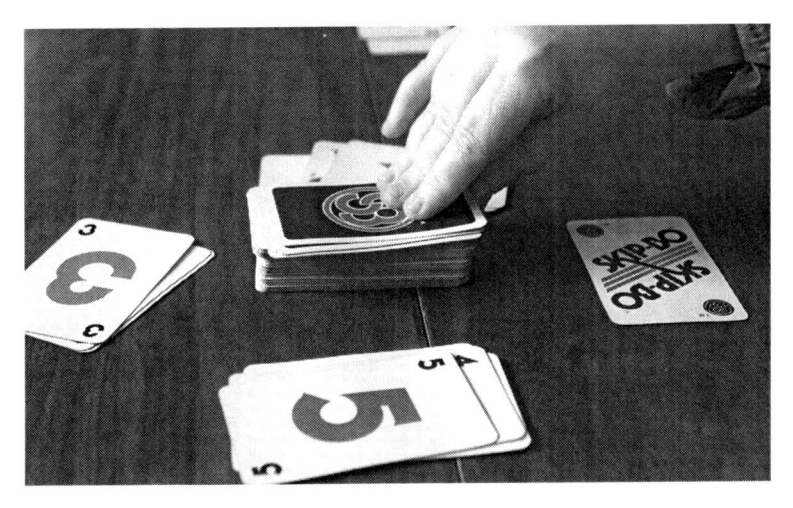

Fig. 5.12 Playing games helps to keep members minds engaged, while providing fodder for conversation

The work of nonprofit management keeps several members busy. "It's put me in a position where I feel like I need to be a leader and I need to keep this club going," says Nick. Work takes a variety of forms, such as writing grants, conducting board meetings, and cleaning the building. Vacuuming is one of the chores Ben undertakes with playfulness. "The attack of the giant vacuum cleaner, Aaahhhhh!" as the roaring machine approaches my camera (Fig. 5.16).

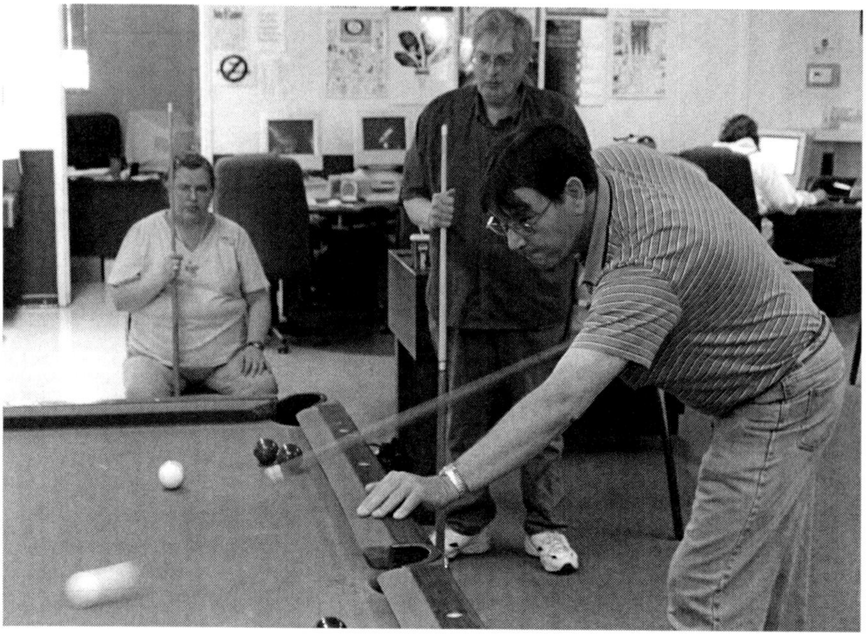

Fig. 5.13 Pool is another popular activity at the P.S. Club. Every Friday members go to the Wellington Recreation Center to play pool for 2 h

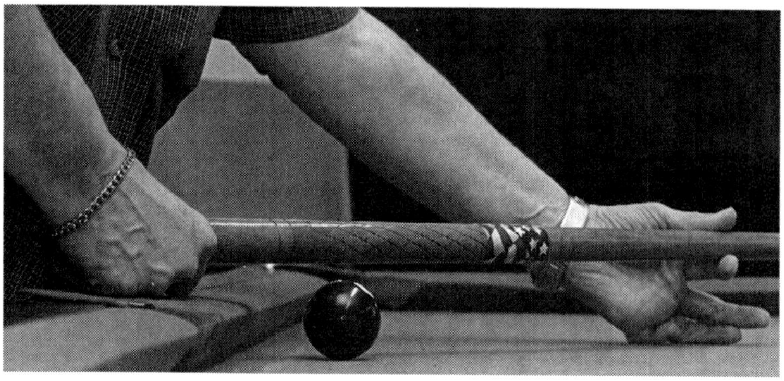

Fig. 5.14 Carl brings his own stick to play pool with other CRO members every Friday. Despite his poor vision and unusual technique, he is an excellent player

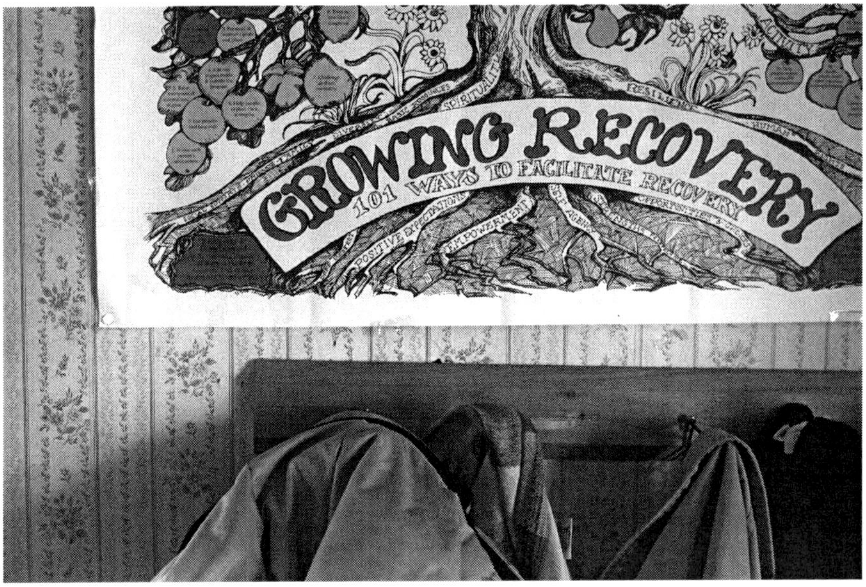

Fig. 5.15 Growing recovery is central to the mission of the P.S. Club

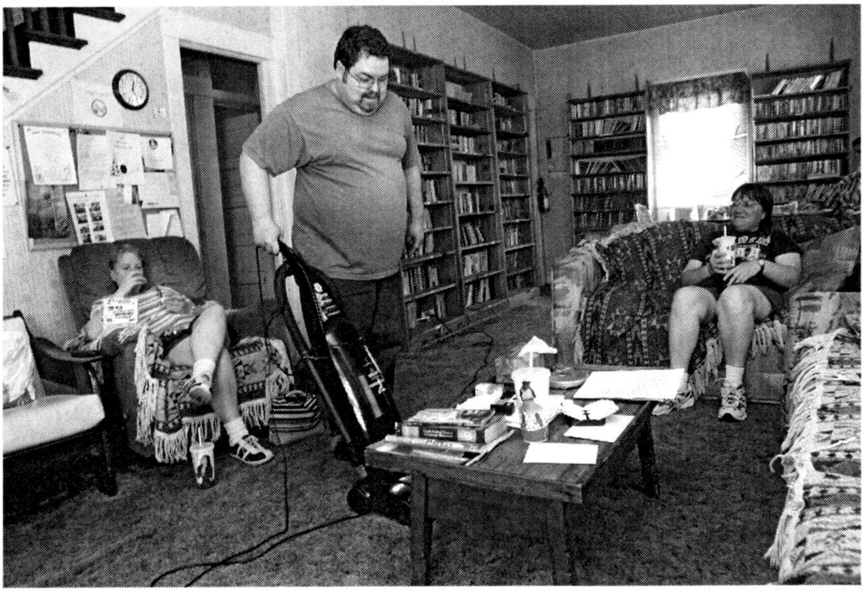

Fig. 5.16 Keeping the P.S. Club clean is a regular chore that members get paid minimum wage to do

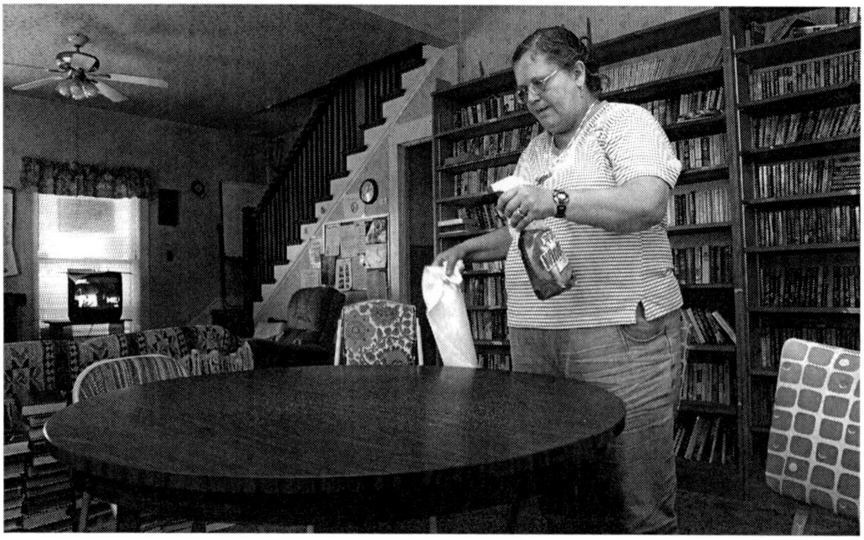

Fig. 5.17 By taking care of the building, members develop a sense of ownership and responsibility for the P.S. Club

By taking on roles and responsibility in the P.S. Club, members learn to fulfill commitments and become leaders. "Some of them will eventually, you know, be willing to take on leadership roles and stuff like that, which gives them a real sense of accomplishment, and makes them feel good about themselves," says Nick.

Being involved has given Mary and others a reason to stay in the community. "I'm just glad to be home and out of that hospital and be able to come to work and be around my friends again you know. Have a normal life," she says (Fig. 5.17).

The club also operates a warm line with peer counseling support. People can call when they want to talk. "Just letting them talk and get their feelings out, cause sometimes that's all people need to do. And then they feel better and they go on," says Nick.

The act of helping others can lead to personal self-revelations and improve self-esteem. "I've done a lot of peer counseling in the last probably 15 years. Finding ways to help me help somebody else has actually helped me too," says Carl.

Although the P.S. Club provides one place where people can feel accepted, members make educational presentations in the community to help all places become understanding and accepting. Nick and Carl made a presentation at local high school where they talked about their own struggles with mental health problems. After recounting several harrowing stories about their own experiences with mental health problems, the presentation turned into a pep talk. "One thing that I want to emphasize with you is that if anything happens with you, don't give up. Just don't give up and say forget it," said Carl. "Keep going. Cause you can be your own best friend or you can be your own worst enemy as well." In the end, the message was simple – mental health problems are challenge to be overcome, much like any other problem humans face (Figs. 5.18 and 5.19).

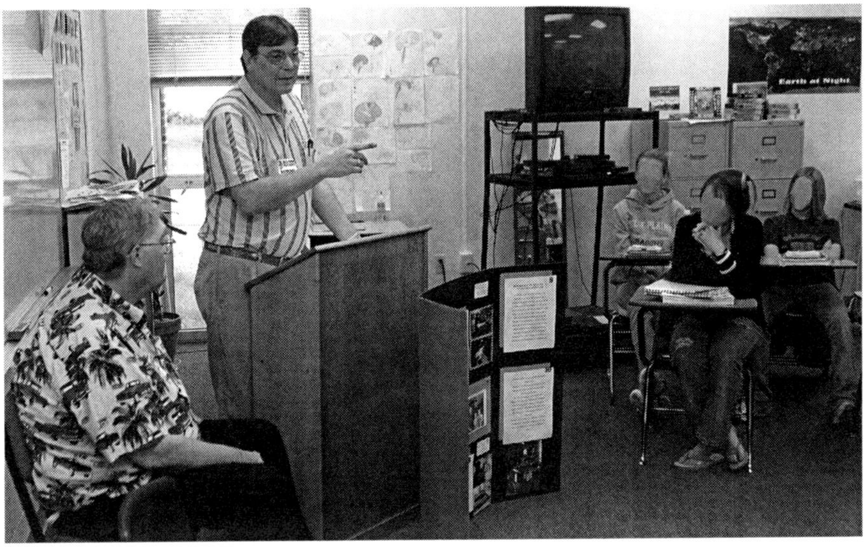

Fig. 5.18 The P.S. Club is always looking for places to make public presentations about mental health problems and the activities of their organization. Pictured here are Carl and Nick presenting to a high school psychology class. The students were brimming with questions, curious about life with mental health problems

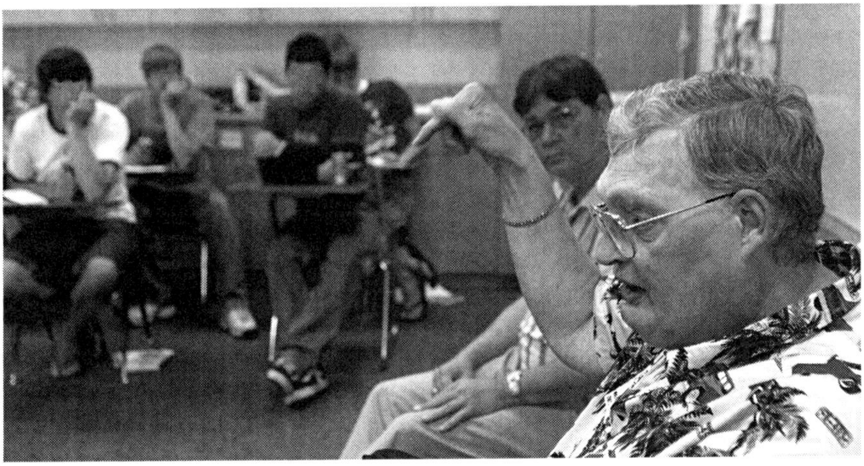

Fig. 5.19 Carl and Nick opened their hearts to the class, sharing both horrifying and heart-warming stories

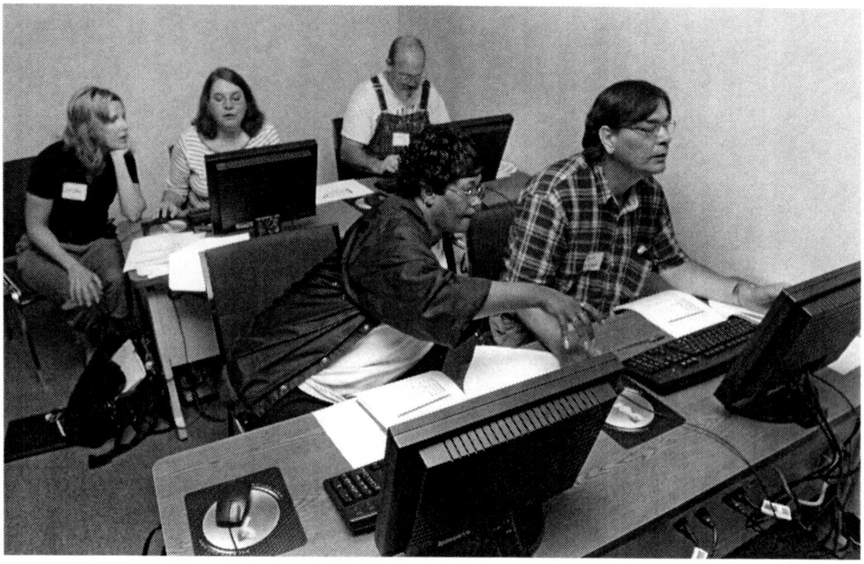

Fig. 5.20 As a state-funded CRO, the P.S. Club receives free technical assistance from the Center for Community Support and Research. Both Carl and Nick attended a computer training organized for CRO leaders

In addition to educating others through presentations, P.S. Club members educate themselves by attending a variety of trainings and conferences (Fig. 5.20). One such conference was the Kansas Recovery Leadership Summit, where participants were given an opportunity to help reform mental health policy. "It's been a very helpful conference because of the fact that we have been able to have the workshops and breakout sessions ourselves," says Carl.

Small group breakout sessions gave people the opportunity to discuss problems and brainstorm solutions for the mental health system. During one of the sessions, Nick recounted one of the problems with a new drug prescription program. "It was like the 200 most popular medications would be covered for like $10 a prescription per month," he says. But the program only covers one or two medications for mental health problems. "So there again, you know, it's a good program but we're left out," he says with frustration.

After refining suggestions made during breakout group discussions everyone voted for the policy changes they found most important. "We're not just attending the workshops or just attending the conference but we're putting ourselves into it as well," says Carl (Fig. 5.21).

One of the strengths of conferences like this one is their ability to bring people together and facilitate networking. "I think all the CROs when we get together like

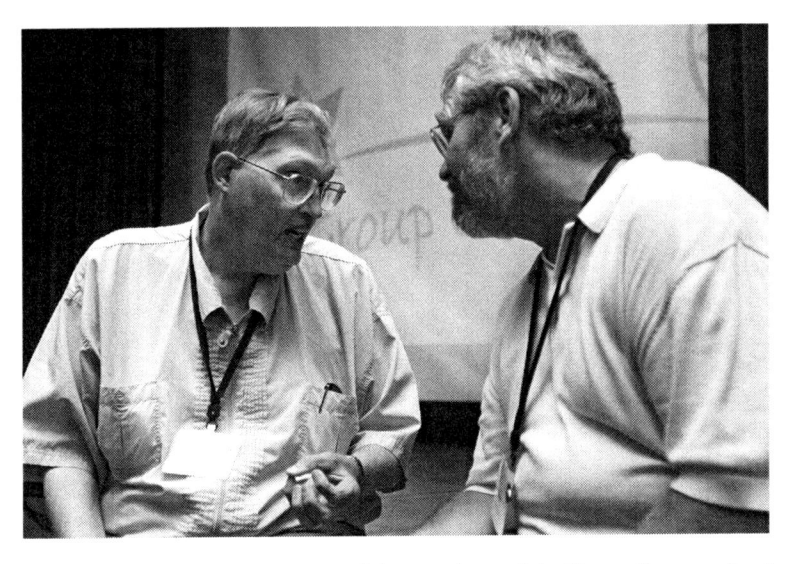

Fig. 5.21 Carl shares his views with one of the organizers of the Kansas Recovery Leadership Summit

that we kinda pump up each other and get more confidence," says Nick. "If one group is doing something that you're not doing right now, it gives you the confidence that you can do that too."

Most everyone sees the conference as a welcome change of pace. "Yeah, I get away from Caldwell for a little while," says Kevin. But to an outsider, the drastic difference between this conference and a regular day can be easily underappreciated. For Kevin, a "regular day, ok, like on a Thursday, I just stay at home and watch TV. And that's all I do," he says.

At the end of the conference, the experience helped people take one more step towards the conference's vision of future where everyone with a mental illness will recover. "We can also learn together how to overcome some of the problems that there are," says Carl.

There are plenty of problems to overcome. Nonprofits operated by people with mental health problems are part of the solution. "Half of your recovery is having those support systems. You know, medication is good but it can only go so far," says Nick.

The social support oriented nonprofits can help people get away from their TVs, out of their homes, and into the community. "It's given me a place to go to so I don't have to sit here and be by myself all day," says Carl.

New relationships can form, social skills can improve, and members can become more outgoing. "If I'm in a store or someplace and somebody from the P.S Club

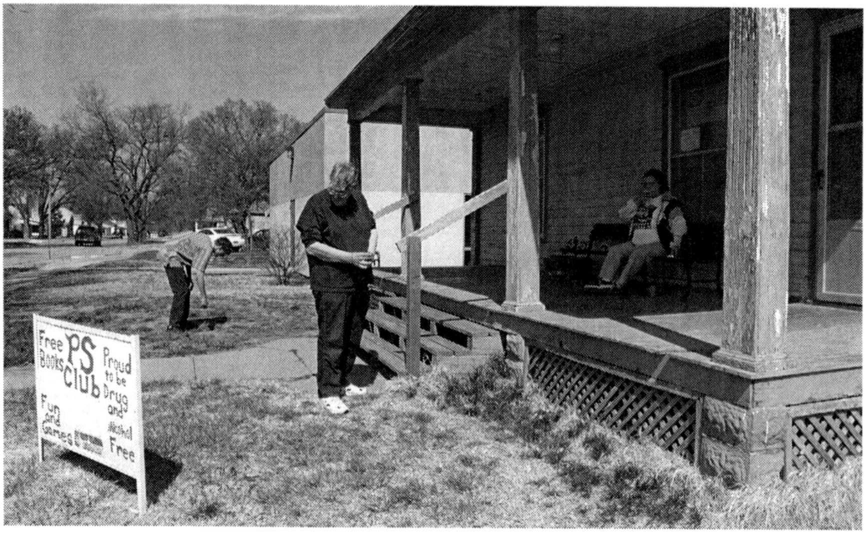

Fig. 5.22 Carl and others helped to pick up trash in the yard of the P.S. Club on a warm winter day. P.S. Club members are responsible for keeping their rental property clean

sees me, they'll always stop and say hello and that's a good feeling. Real good feeling," says Carl.

Members can transition away from the dependency roles that consumers typically hold and into wellness-enhancing helper roles. "If I can help other people, it's satisfying to me and makes me feel good," says Nick. Involvement in the organizations daily operations is another way to contribute. "Working here has helped a lot too, with self-esteem," says Carl (Fig. 5.22).

The fact that everyone including the director has mental health problems helps to create an understanding atmosphere (Figs. 5.23 and 5.24). "People are just more comfortable when they feel like someone really understands how they feel and what they went through and everything," says Nick.

When people feel comfortable, they stay long enough to make friends and get involved in organizational operations. "That's something else I don't want to see change is the feeling of being wanted there," says Carl.

Members can find a new appreciation for their life. "Me going to this club, I've been able to appreciate the life that I have, even though I go through a lot of pain," says Laura, who recently started attending. Hope for the future can grow strong, which Mary cherishes. "Right now I feel like a brand new person," she says.

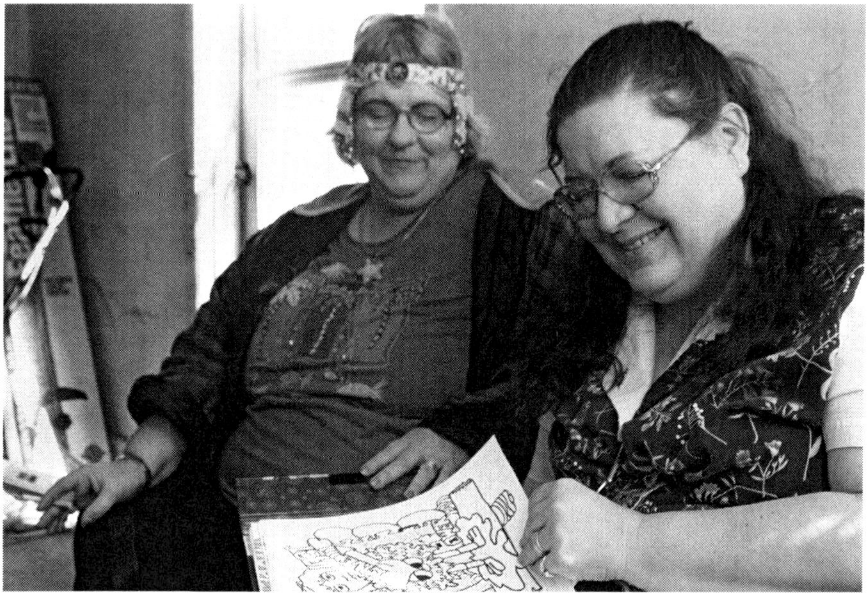

Fig. 5.23 The P.S. Club is a place where people share not only stories and feelings but also creative endeavors such as these drawings

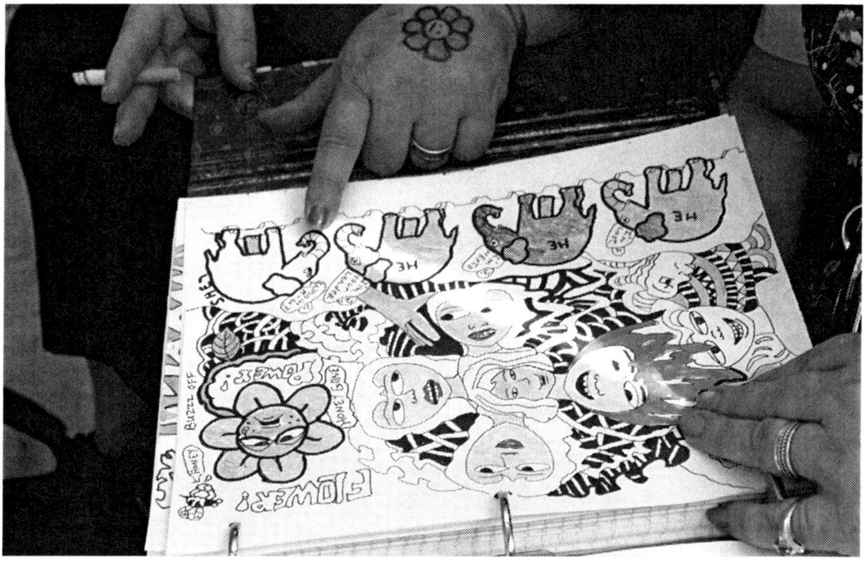

Fig. 5.24 Creative expression can serve as an important emotional outlet for people with mental health problems

Mary's Story

"Don't worry about it, you won't get pregnant." Bad advice, especially when it comes from a teenage boy without birth control. At the age of 17, Mary learned the hard way. She dropped out of high school and had a baby.

After her son was born Mary had a mental breakdown. For two years doctors called it mental fatigue from the pregnancy. But Mary had been showing signs of schizophrenia for years. At one point she told her mother, "'MOM, A devil is in the closet!'

> She said, 'WHAT?'
> 'There's a devil in the closet.'
> 'How can you tell?'
> 'Well he's red and he's got a long nose and long red finger nails and long toe nails.'

'Honey that's not the devil, there's nothing but nothing in there'," her mother explained to Mary. "Then I'd hallucinate, I'd think that was a séance or something and somebody was gonna come back from their grave and haunt me. This all went on the time I was 5–17. Then, after [my son] was born, it got worse."

At the age of 19, Mary was diagnosed with paranoid schizophrenia. She spent the next 9 years of her life in and out of the Arkansas State Hospital. "Mom was taking care of [my son]. Her and my step dad and [my son] came up and seen me at least every 2 weeks and I got to go home some weekends. Last time I went up there I was up there for 8 months and that's when I got my G.E.D. I was working on my G.E.D. every time I would go to Little Rock."

From Little Rock, Mary moved to Belle Plaine, Kansas, to live in a trailer near her dad. While there, she worked in a sheltered workshop for 5 years as a ceramic assistant. Unfortunately this period of relative job stability did not translate into a period of mental stability. "I was a regular at St. Joe [a nearby psychiatric hospital], at least for 8 or 10 years," she says.

Fundamental to breaking her hospitalization cycle was Clozaril, a second-generation antipsychotic medication. In the 14 years that she has been on it, she has only been hospitalized seven times. Clozaril is not the perfect drug, however, and Mary is dependent on many other drugs to manage her symptoms. She takes Neurontin for mood regulation and anxiety, Klonopin for anxiety and to help her sleep at night, Zoloft for depression, Detrol for an overactive bladder, laxatives and FiberCon are for the constipating side effects of the other drugs. The balance is delicate and experimentation with other medications that might work better can be dangerous. One of Mary's more recent hospitalizations was the result of a disastrous change in her anxiety medication. "I went flat berserk," Mary says. "I got sick over night. I couldn't even stand up or walk or do nothing."

Mary's dependence on drugs and the prescription decisions of her doctors is tremendous. She attributes most of her well-being (or lack thereof) to her medications. With little direct control over her mental health, Mary looks to mental health professionals for advice on what to do and how to live. Fortunately, they frequently give her good advice but her compliant and submissive nature does also get her into trouble.

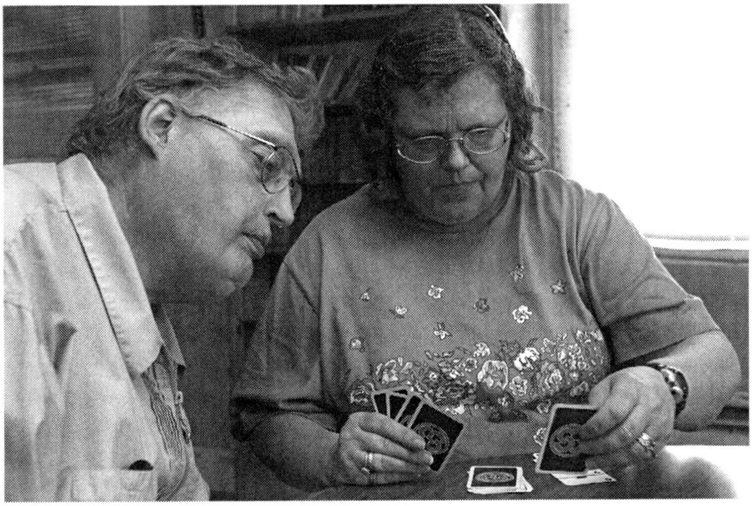

Mary's Story

Fig. 5.25 When playing cards, Mary sometimes struggles to figure out how to best play her cards. Other members, such as Carl, frequently offer their assistance

Mary's tendency towards deferral has led her into a number of problematic romantic relationships. Her first boyfriend was not interested in raising the baby she had after he told her she would not get pregnant. Her first husband remarried and had kids while she was in a psychiatric hospital. Her second marriage was an abusive one. "He beat me up really bad 1 day and I was trying to get out the door, and he grabbed my radio and I ran to the door and he chased me down about two stairs and he tripped me on my face with his foot and he started kicking me."

While Mary does get pushed around sometimes, she always stands up for herself when she knows something is wrong. She immediately divorced her abusive husband and pressed charges. "I was bruised from head to toe and he had to go to court and they got him for abuse and resisting arrest and domestic violence," she says. Mary has a strong sense of fairness and prides herself on being a good-natured and honest citizen. "Well, I try to get along with people. I try to keep my job and do everything I'm supposed to at my job. Try to help people as much as I can and I do have mental problems." It is often Mary's confusion that leads her to defer to others. Sometimes she just doesn't know what to do. "My train of thought … isn't too good. I'm taking Neurontin for that," she explains. "I try to say something … seems like I go off the subject and come around to something else." This mental confusion can make relating to others difficult. Mary's self-esteem and sense of adequacy suffer as a result of her problems (Fig. 5.25).

At the P.S. Club, Mary finds patience for her problems and this helps her work to overcome them. Nick, the director, is always accommodating. "[Nick] says, 'if you need to go to the doctor don't worry about it. We'll find someone to take your place.' He says, 'just do what you can.'" Mary continues, "Anytime you tell him anything he listens to you. Some people just say I don't have time to hear your problems. He doesn't laugh at us. He doesn't make fun of us."

Mary was one of the first members of the P.S. Club, participating back in 1986 when it was still part of the Sumner Mental Health Center. For many years her participation was sporadic. "When I was taking Stelazine I wasn't hardly involved in the group at all. I wouldn't get out of my apartment. I was too paranoid, too nervous," she says. "Until about 2 years after I got on Clozaril that I started trying to socialize at the P.S. Club." Mary comes to the P.S. Club to see her friends and "to keep from being lonely and not by myself and stuff. I come up here and eat lunch and play cards or sit on the front porch (Figs. 5.26 and 5.27)."

When she became more involved she started working as a shift manager, which has provided her with some extra spending money. "I do my chores, which include emptying the ice trays, cleaning the bathroom, washing off the table and chairs, taking out the trash, washing the white leather chair…Let's see, I can't remember, I think that's about all I do." In addition to her shift manager work she is the treasurer of the P.S. Club. "I have to sign the checks before [Nick] can cash any," says Mary. "I have to sign the checks for payroll and I sign the checks for supplies. I sign the checks for gas and stuff like that."

The familiar, accepting, and flexible work environment has allowed Mary to maintain employment at the P.S. Club for 12 years, longer than any other job she has had in the past. "There are more people here that understand what you're going through, people you can talk to," she says.

The work helps Mary maintain healthy levels of stress. "I just have to keep myself motivated to stay busy and do things so I won't think about all those thoughts that come back from the past." Staying busy is actually fundamental to Mary's mental health (Fig. 5.28). "I have to stay busy. I'll have to keep my mind concentrated

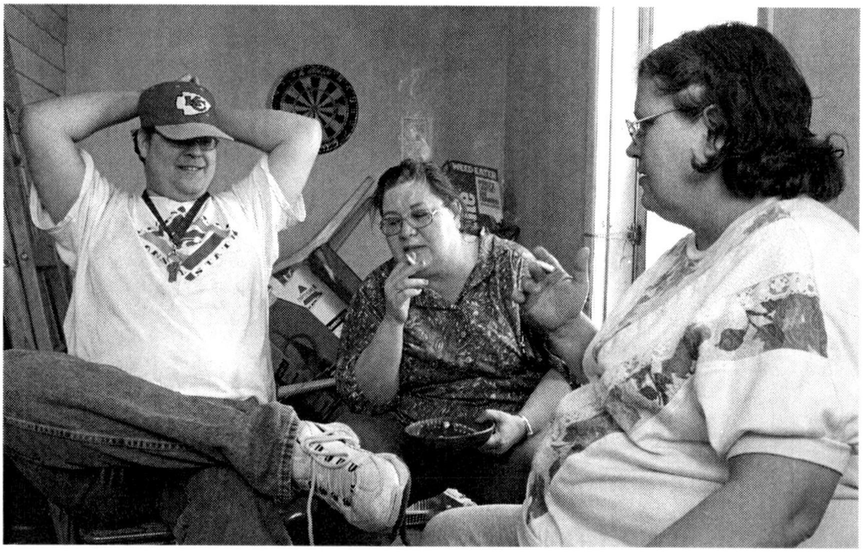

Fig. 5.26 Conversation at the P.S. Club is intermittent. At times, everyone is engaged and enjoying themselves

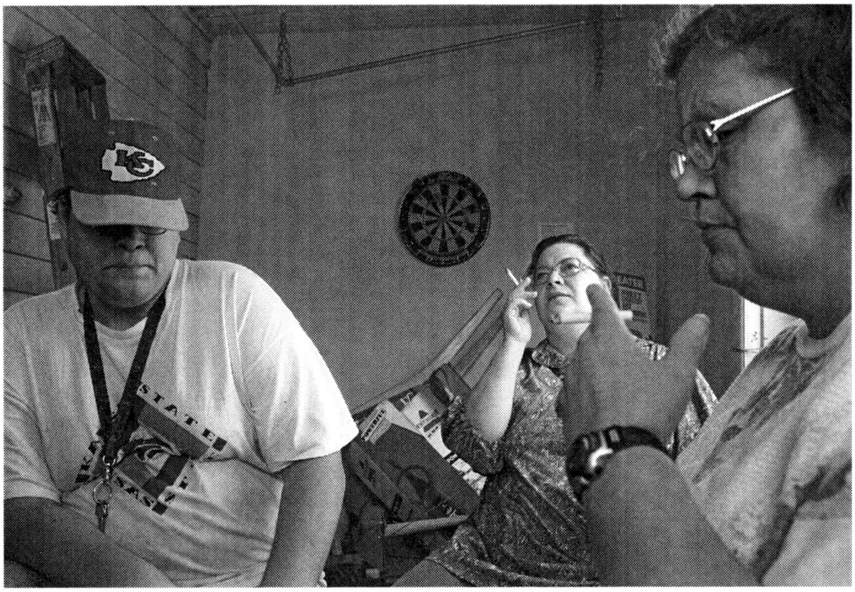

Mary's Story

Fig. 5.27 Conversation at the P.S. Club is not always easy or abundant. It is not uncommon for the room to fall silent, leaving members to their own thoughts

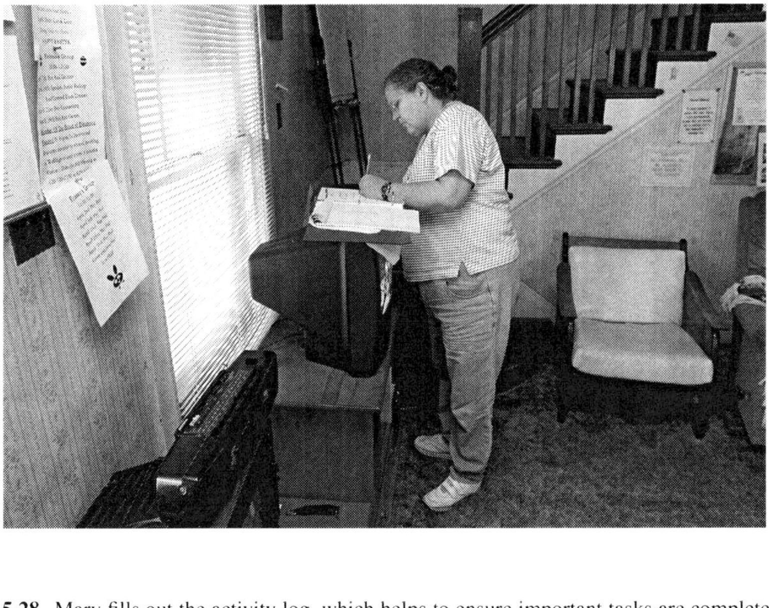

Fig. 5.28 Mary fills out the activity log, which helps to ensure important tasks are completed on a regular basis

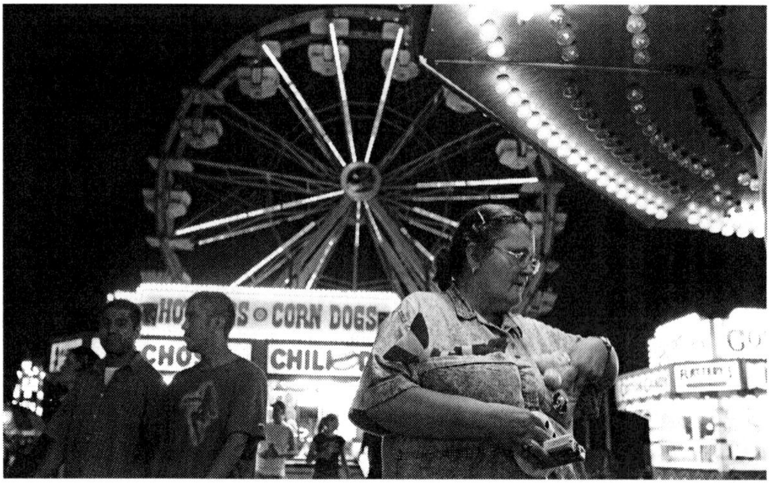

Fig. 5.29 Mary attended a fair with Carl. They played several games and came home with pockets full of stuffed animals

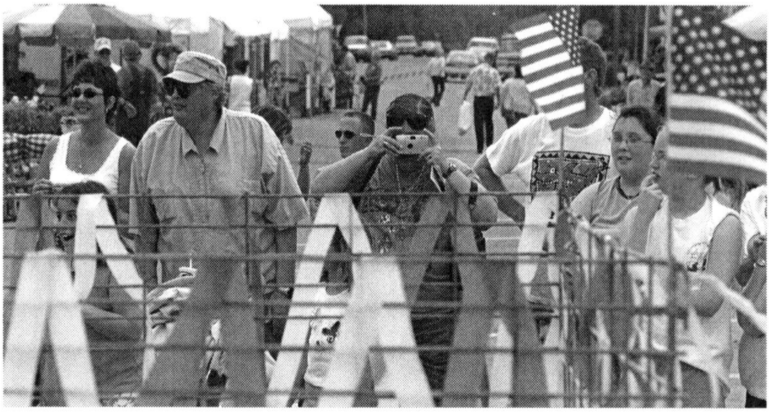

Fig. 5.30 Mary takes a picture of a passing float at a parade near Wellington. Parades are a big draw in the small towns of Kansas. Mary and Carl are regular attendees

on something, doing something everyday. If I don't I could easily end up in the state hospital." Boredom allows her to dwell on her problems and develop paranoia. The P.S. Club engages Mary in something productive that helps others.

Despite her problems, Mary is satisfied with her life and many aspects of it bring her pride, including her family, her competencies, and her job. "I'm proud that I'm able to go out into the community without people saying, 'Look at her! She's mentally retarded,'" she says. "I'm proud that [Nick] has his confidence in me to be a treasurer." Today Mary feels that she is doing better than ever before (Figs. 5.29 and 5.30). Her recovery journey is long and arduous but there is hope. "My strengths? Fighting schizophrenia," she says.

Nick's Story

Nick knew mental health problems before he knew puberty. "I started thinking I seen angels flying around at 10 years old" he says. He also knew he should keep it a secret. "I didn't really tell anybody about it because my great uncle, he thought he was a prophet and he had preached that he seen different things. Everybody said he was crazy so I didn't share that with anybody."

While the hallucinations were odd, they weren't scary and did not cause major disruptions in Nick's life. Nick lived a relatively normal childhood with two loving parents, an older brother and a younger sister. More troubling was a persistently timid disposition that dates back to his years as a toddler. "They just thought I was just shy, they didn't realize that it could be a mental illness." When his parents friends came over Nick said he "would hide and kinda peek around the door but I would never come out. I guess I was just real paranoid then."

As Nick progressed through adolescence and into adulthood his schizophrenic symptoms became progressively worse, although he was unaware of it at the time. Time sequences would become distorted and Nick would know what someone was going to say before they said it. "I'd heard things and stuff like that before but it wasn't a constant thing. And I'd always think, 'well, probably just got a little ESP or something. I kinda categorized it as that and went on,' " he recalls.

In 1974, Nick graduated from high school with 2 years of experience working as a machinist. He continued his work while attending Northern Oklahoma University and in 1977 he received his associate's degree in accounting. Unfortunately, by this point in time his symptoms had worsened and Nick grew increasingly shy. "I was so introverted you know, and that showed when I was talking to people," he says. "I think they felt like this guy is not really confident in himself, we don't really need him. I really think that's what kept me from getting a job in that field."

Machinist jobs were easier to come by and he already had experience in the field, so Nick decided to make a career of it, albeit a rather haphazard one. "I switched jobs all the time. I'd always get to thinking they was messing me around some way or another," he says. "I figured it up like 17 different places in 17 years. Of course there were some times at the end there that I wouldn't be working for a few months here and there."

To combat shyness, Nick resorted to drinking. "One thing I used to do in my late teens and early twenties was a lot of drinking," he says. "Of course that was before I realized that I was mentally ill and back then I was so backwards and shy. That's really the only time I corresponded with many people at all, is when I had been drinking."

Substance abuse helped Nick meet his first wife, who also had a taste for intoxication. Together they had three boys in the 4 years they were married. When they divorced, Nick's wife preferred a life of parties and drugs to the responsibilities of parenting. "She told the judge that she felt like I was the better parent and that she didn't want the responsibility and that's the way we did it," explains Nick.

Nick faced a formidable challenge raising three kids by himself, two of which were in diapers. To make ends meet, he also had to work 50–60 h a week. The stress made his mental health problems worse and his hallucinations became frightening. "I had a hallucination where Jesus had punched me right in the face!" he said. "I thought to myself, 'man, I must be a terrible person for him to hit me in the face like that.' What's weird about these hallucinations is that you feel the pain. It's not just like watching TV or anything. You will feel the pain and that's what convinces you that it's really real."

His children also suffered from the situation. "I went to work, I'd come home and I'd fall asleep on the couch. I wouldn't wake up till the next day," says Nick. In addition to exhaustion, the hallucinations interfered with his parenting. "I'd go to the grocery store and buy my groceries, then I'd be afraid to eat them, afraid they was gonna poison me," Nick explains. "Luckily at that time, this was before I moved in with my parents, my oldest son was old enough that he would get around and make him and his brothers something to eat."

Nick faced this situation for 5 years before suffering a complete mental breakdown. "I went to work the next morning and everything just completely had changed. I forgot how to do my job the way I needed to do it," he says. The world became a blur. "I thought all kinds of things were going on and all I was really doing was sitting there staring at the wall," says Nick. "In my mind I was doing a lot of things, a lot of crazy things."

After 3 months, Nick finally got some help. "Even though there's been mental illness in the family and everything, my parents or nobody stopped to think that I could be having mental problems," says Nick. Along with not thinking about it was the fact that mental health problems were not something to be talked about. Without discussion, there is no understanding. For Nick, the stigma and ignorance surrounding mental health problems prevented him from receiving treatment for the first 15 years he spent as an adult with schizophrenia.

After his breakdown, Nick and his kids moved in with Nick's parents. "I felt bad that it got to where I couldn't function on my own and I had to live with them," Nick remembers. But Nick doesn't remember much else because he was so intensely confused. An entire year of his life is simply missing.

In 1989, Nick started taking Thorazine to treat his symptoms. "Even though it didn't work real good, when I started with the Thorazine, within about 3 or 4 days I could see a big difference. At least I got a hold of a little bit of reality there," Nick remembers. "It was enough to keep me out of trouble." Unfortunately, tolerances were built, doses were increased, and eventually doctors were forced to switch to a new medication. The cycle repeated itself and Nick experienced a variety of nasty side effects. "People could tell something was wrong real obvious, cause of the way Prolixin did ya," he says. "My joints all tightened up and I kinda walked like this [walks like a zombie]. Everywhere I went, it was just terrible."

Terrible, but still better than when he had the breakdown. Nick re-entered the world with a reduced level of stress because of his disengagement during the breakdown. He discovered that stress levels had a major impact on the intensity of his symptoms. "Schizophrenia is something that is always there but stress can really bring it out," he says. "I can do about anything I want to, for a little while, but once I start getting stressed I gotta quit for a while or my thinking and everything is not clear."

Over time, Nick learned to regulate himself, taking on new things slowly and taking breaks whenever the stress piled up. Soon after he started feeling better, he moved out of his parents' home to live by himself. Over the next 2 years, Nick slowly had his kids move back in with him, one at a time.

His newfound understanding of how stress impacted his symptoms provided insight into his unstable employment history. Although he didn't realize it at the time, the breaks he took between jobs may have been the stress relief he desperately needed to prevent a complete breakdown. The job Nick held when his breakdown occurred was the best he ever had. His boss was promising high-paying promotions. "I worked there longer than I worked anywhere in my life and I had a complete breakdown," he says. "It's like before I'd always gave myself a break, 2 or 3 months here, 2 or 3 months there, and I think the stress just built up to the point where it caused a complete breakdown that time."

Two years after being put on antipsychotics, Nick started attending the P.S. Club. Reluctant at first, Nick was coaxed into going by his case manager. "She started coming by my house visiting with me and talking with me and it actually took her 3 or 4 months before she could talk me in to attending P.S. Club at the Mental Health Center," he says. His reluctance was partially due to shyness but attending the club also forced him to accept his identity as someone with mental health problems. "I was really battling with myself, just the idea that I was mentally ill. Kept trying to convince myself that they made a mistake and this and that even though the medicine was helping," he says. "That's why I realized a lot of the time with people, it takes time and it's hard sometimes to get them to start. Once I started though, it wasn't 2 or 3 months and I really liked it then. I was looking forward to going" (Fig. 5.31).

At the time, the P.S. Club was a psychosocial club in the mental health center. The club focused on organizing recreational and social activities with the idea that social interaction is therapeutic. The psychosocial club was controlled by mental health professionals, however.

After 2 years as a regular member of the P.S. Club, Nick was encouraged by his therapist to write a grant to the Kansas Social and Rehabilitation Services to start the P.S. Club as a consumer run organization. With his parenting situation under control, Nick decided to take on the challenge. In 1993, with $16,000, the P.S. Club opened its doors as an independent nonprofit, the fifth CRO in Kansas.

Nick struggled from the beginning to find help. Other consumers lost interest after 3 days of grant writing and nobody was a reliable transportation provider the way Nick was. It wasn't long before he took primary responsibility for the club. The role of director was ingrained into his behavior and he became the P.S. Club's charismatic leader. In the beginning, all work was unpaid. Grant money went towards rent, utilities, and transportation. Despite its voluntary workforce, the P.S. Club was able to operate 40 h per week.

Three years after its initiation, the P.S. Club's budget was increased and people started getting paid for some of the work they were doing, albeit below minimum wage.

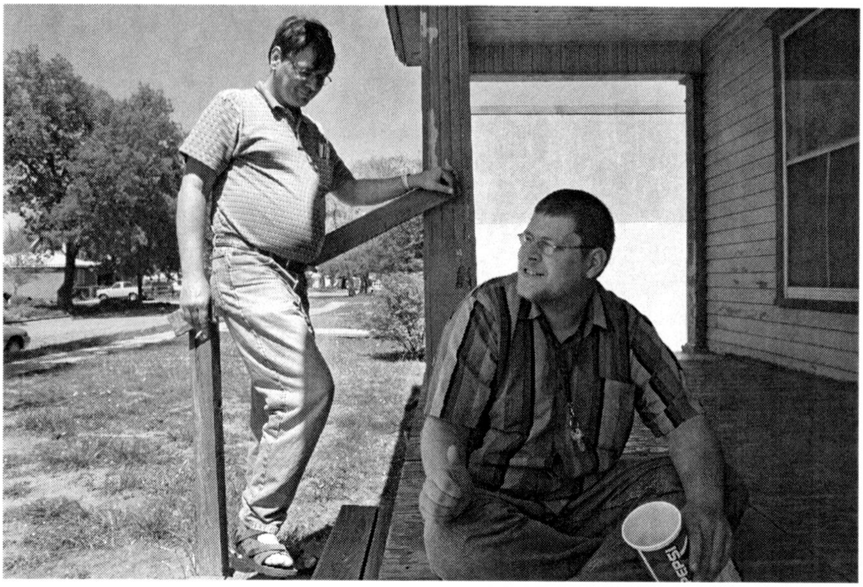

Fig. 5.31 Nick smiles at a joke as he walks towards the entrance of the P.S. Club. One of the draws of the porch is that you can keep track of all the people coming and going

The income was a nice boost for Nick, although he couldn't make too much without losing his Social Security Disability Income benefits (Fig. 5.32).

That same year Nick's medication was switched to Clozaril, a second-generation antipsychotic medication. Vivid changes in Nick's symptoms occurred. "I think about what my mother told me when I got on Clozaril. I'd been on Clozaril for about a month. She says, 'You know, I see that gleem in your eye that I haven't seen since you was a little boy,'" he says. "But that is how much it affected me, the Clozaril did. It was the first one that really got me close to normal, where I was naturally happy."

Nick saw a tremendous reduction in his level of paranoia. As a result, his shyness dissipated. Dormant social skills rapidly emerged. "I wasn't very talkative, near as much talkative with the family members until I got on Clozaril," he says. "When I went to my high school class reunion, 30 year reunion, that's the first time I had went to one and I had a really good time," he says. "I didn't struggle with the social stuff like I used to. I felt real comfortable talking to everybody. It went real well."

The side effects were better too. No movement disorders. Clozaril isn't perfect, though. "Something that irritates the heck out of me but it's something that I gotta put up with. Every night when I go to sleep, you know how when you go to sleep your saliva glands usually quit working. Well, mine don't quit working and when I wake up the next morning my pillow is soaked from slobbering all night," he says. "Another side effect is weight gain. I was pretty lucky that I'd been really skinny my whole life or I could of got really huge taking the Clozaril." Although medication has cleared Nick's thinking, he still has to be

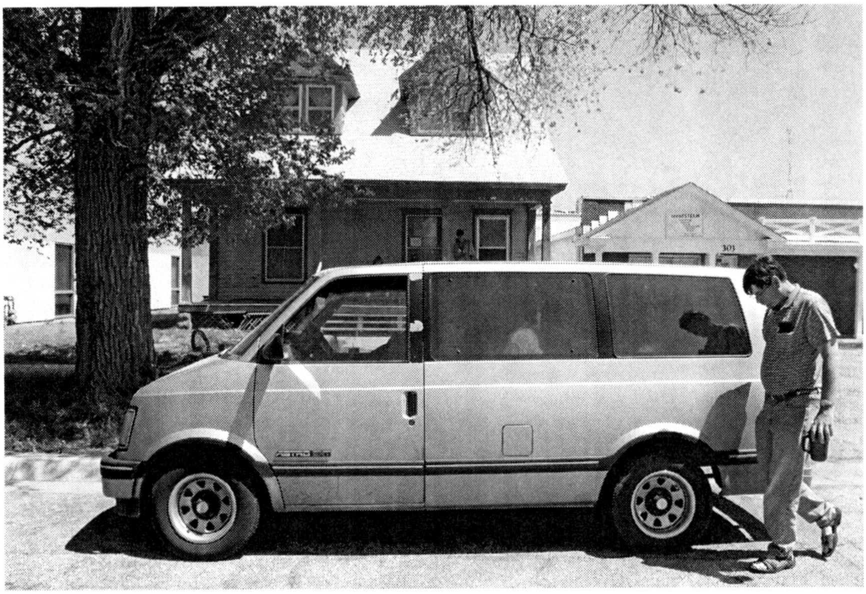

Fig. 5.32 On Mondays, Wednesdays, and Fridays Nick provides everyone with transportation to and from the club. He spends over 4 h behind the wheel each of these days, driving people all over Sumner County

careful. "Even with medication and still up to now, I can't put myself under an excessive amount of stress. Stress will mess me up quicker than anything," he says. "If I get to feeling too stressed, which makes it nice about this job, I just put everything back for a couple of days and just relax until I get to feeling better." The flexible and understanding work environment of the P.S. Club is critical to his success (Fig. 5.33).

Involvement in the P.S. Club's recreational activities is another strategy Nick uses to manage his stress. "It helps me just coming up and being with other people and socializing and playing games and stuff, gets my mind off of everything," he says. While Nick still enjoys the recreational activities at the club, he doesn't have as much time for them now as he used to. As funding for the club increased, so did the paperwork and the number of administrative responsibilities. In the beginning, Nick's primary responsibility was providing transportation. Today, grants and quarterly reports are more complicated. Taxes and payroll must be filed. Quarterly meetings for CRO leaders across the state must be attended.

The activities of the P.S. Club have also diversified. Presentations about mental health problems are now being made in churches and schools (Fig. 5.34). A newsletter is mailed out every month. A peer counseling warm line has been established. "I have one lady, she calls me about every week or two you know and she just wants to talk to somebody for 5 or 10 min and then she's fine for another couple of weeks," says Nick.

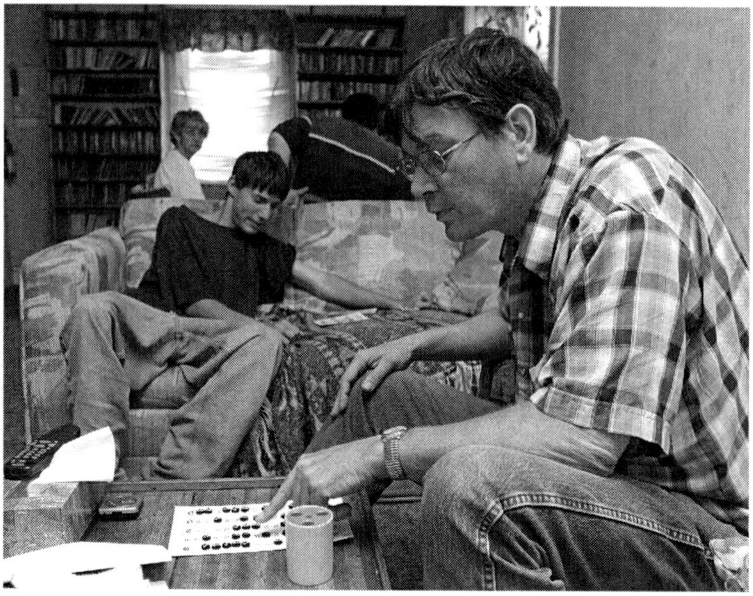

Fig. 5.33 As executive director, Nick frequently plays the role of activity organizer. Pictured here he reads off bingo numbers while everyone waits in anticipation

"She's usually not having a lot of problems at the time she's just lonely. Sometimes that's all it takes with people, someone that will be there for them and listen to them and let them air their feelings out so they can get to feeling better."

Outside of his involvement in the P.S. Club is his involvement at church, which he attends every Sunday with his girlfriend. Religion has always been important to him, although his faith was tested during his breakdown. "I felt like I was really tested for a while. I could remember 'Oh God why did you let this happen to me?'" he says. Today Nick feels like maybe the purpose behind his mental health problems was to start the P.S. Club. "He put me in the position and gave me the knowledge to get the club started and there's a lot of people that's benefited by my hard work. Maybe that's the purpose."

Throughout Nick's recovery, he has become increasingly independent. Instead of being dependent on his parents for basic care, he now visits them on holidays and talks on the phone with them regularly as friends. A similar transformation has occurred in his relationship with his therapist. Initially, Nick was a mental patient receiving therapy. Over time, the relationship has not faded but transitioned into one of colleague, as both are employed by the government to help people with mental health problems. The money Nick makes as director of the P.S. Club has helped him become financially independent.

Fig. 5.34 Nick shares stories about his struggles with schizophrenia and his path towards recovery with high-school students during a presentation about mental health problems by the P.S. Club

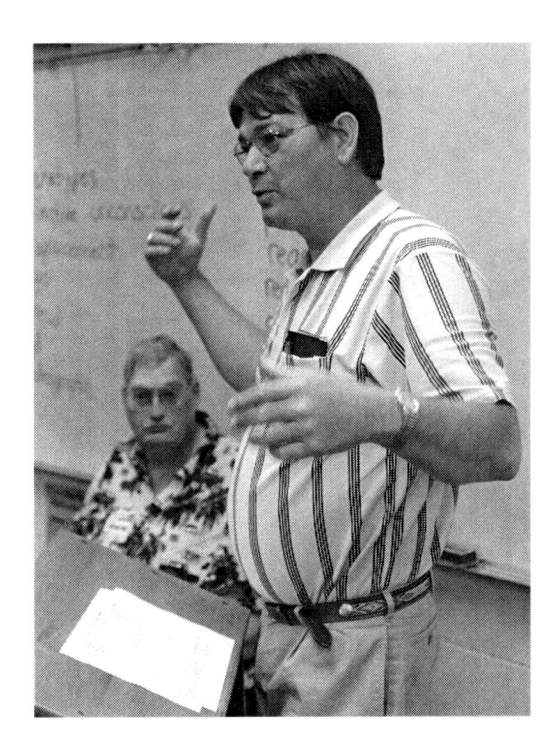

As director, he has also developed many skills. "I've gotten a lot better at talking to other people especially in public speaking. I'm not near as nervous and stuff as I used to be when I do presentations," he says. "By working for the club I've kinda brought back a lot of the accounting and stuff that I did in college." Nick has also become generally more responsible because he has to turn so many things around in a timely manner.

Many members, such as John, have come to see Nick as a role model. "Even though he has a mental illness like I do, he is able to do what he does as director," says John. "That has been encouraging to me, to know that I can do more than I think I can." Long-time member Mary agrees. "We all respect him. We all get along real good. Anytime you tell him anything, he listens to you," says Mary.

A primary motivator in Nick's work is the sense of satisfaction he receives when helping others. "If I can keep it goin' and get the paperwork done and everything and help all these people have a place to come, that's gratifying to me," he says. "Lord knows I'm not makin' much money doin' it. You gotta do it because you wanna help people." Nick helps all the P.S. Club members and all the P.S. Club members help Nick. "Sometimes I need these people just as much as they need me," he says (Fig. 5.35).

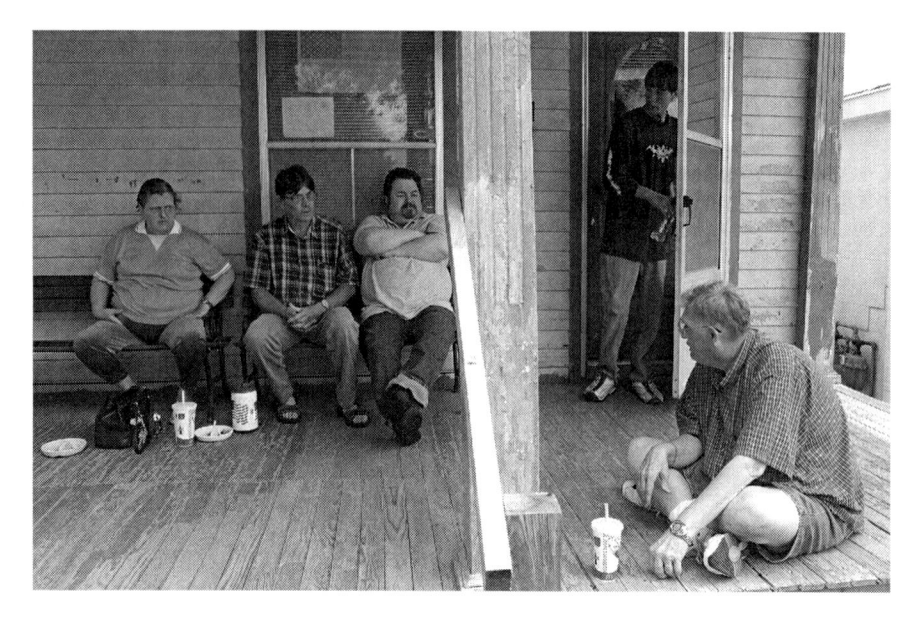

Fig. 5.35 The P.S. Club is an important social outlet for Nick. Pictured here he spends time talking with other members of the club

Carl's Story

Carl knew hate before he knew love. "My dad would come home from work and the first thing he'd do is head for the leather strap. 'Come here' and I hadn't done anything," Carl remembers. His father's criticism was relentless. "I was out cleaning snow off of different parts of the drive-way or whatever. Every time my father walked by, he made some sort of snide sarcastic remark about the way I picked it up, the way I scooped it, the way I shoveled it, the way I threw it!" Carl quickly learned what his dad taught him. "I'm worthless. I'm no good. I can't do anything right. I'll never amount to anything," he says. Low self-esteem became a defining quality of his personality.

Despite the abuse, Carl was a good student in school. However, he was not successful socially. "I didn't really have any friends outside of school. Although I rode in a car pool, I still didn't get along with those guys," he remembers. "Yeah, I didn't joke very much. I didn't have a lot of fun like some kids did."

Making life more difficult was the discovery of two brain tumors at the age of 19 and 24. Their removal came at a price. "All I have is half of one eye. The tumors damaged my optical nerves," he says. "I also had to have radiation to deaden out any tissue that was left over that they couldn't remove."

The damage left him unable to pursue his career interests in printing and graphic arts. "I had to give all that up because without peripheral vision, without any depth perception, it's dangerous to be around the machinery," he says.

"To do the graphic work you have to use Exacto knives and I don't want to accidentally cut off a finger."

Two years after surgery, unable to find a job, Carl ended up in Topeka State Hospital. "I kept saying 'I don't need help' and after I got in there I found out how much help I needed," he remembers. While there he was diagnosed with major depression. "I was actually scared when they first diagnosed me because I didn't know what the illness was, what it would do to me, or how people would react to me when they found out that I had that problem," Carl says. Over the next 10 years Carl spent as much time in the hospital as out of it. "I'd been in and out so much they put a revolving door on my room," he jokes.

After leaving the hospital, Carl stayed in Topeka to get away from his father. While there he got involved in Breakthrough House, a drop-in center that follows the Fountain House model. The model holds values similar to those of the P.S. Club, except it is controlled by nonconsumers. Carl's experiences at Breakthrough House helped him start to make significant gains towards recovery. For the first time in his life he had close friends.

Carl got married for the first time in 1993. Unfortunately he didn't marry the right person and in 1997 he moved from Topeka to Caldwell to get away from her. "I got tired of my wife lying to me, cheating on me, and stealing from me," he says.

It was in Caldwell that Carl started occasionally attending the P.S. Club. Introduced by a friend, Carl developed many more friendships at the club and started attending regularly. Much of his improved mood is attributed to his participation in the P.S. Club. "It's given me a place to go to so I don't have to sit at home and be by myself all day," he says. "I can go and be with other people." The active involvement helps to prevent stagnant rumination on negative thoughts (Fig. 5.36).

His close friendships make him feel important. "I've told [Nick] things that I wouldn't tell anybody else or he has told me things that he wouldn't tell anybody else," he says. "That's a good feeling to be able to talk to somebody like that, and know that they trust you also. That makes me feel pretty good." Even P.S. Club acquaintances are meaningful. "If I'm in a store or someplace and somebody from the P.S Club sees me, they'll always stop and say hello and that's a good feeling. Real good feeling," he says.

In 1999, Carl moved to Wellington and started working as a shift manager at the P.S. Club. "I'm more involved in the P.S. Club than I was with Breakthrough House," he says. "Working here has helped a lot with self-esteem." His work at the P.S. Club is also personally meaningful. "I had swept it and scrubbed it. I did it because I wanted to, not that I felt that it was something I had to do but I did it cause I wanted to," he says. "Going to the [Center for Community Support & Research] meetings with [Nick], I wanna do that. Going to make presentations, I wanna do that" (Fig. 5.37).

While Carl has made tremendous strides toward recovery in the past 15 years, he still has a long way to go (Fig. 5.38). Impatience and anger remain problems at times. "I sometimes get impatient when other people take too long to do something I think they could have done quicker. My anger flares up sometimes," he says.

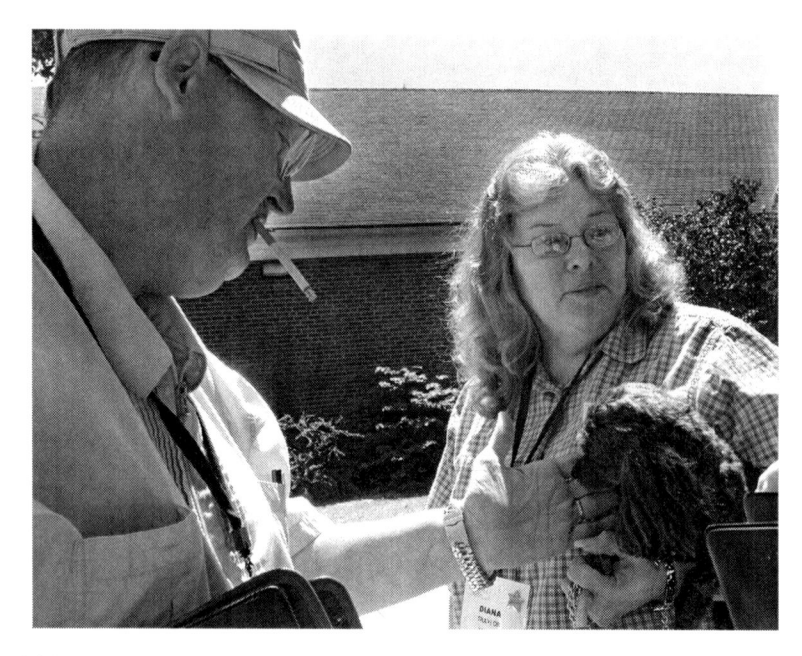

Fig. 5.36 As a member of the P.S. Club, Carl attended the Kansas Recovery Leadership Summit at Wichita State University. He loves these conferences because he gets to meet new people from across the state. Pictured here he takes a moment to pet the dog of a fellow conference attendee

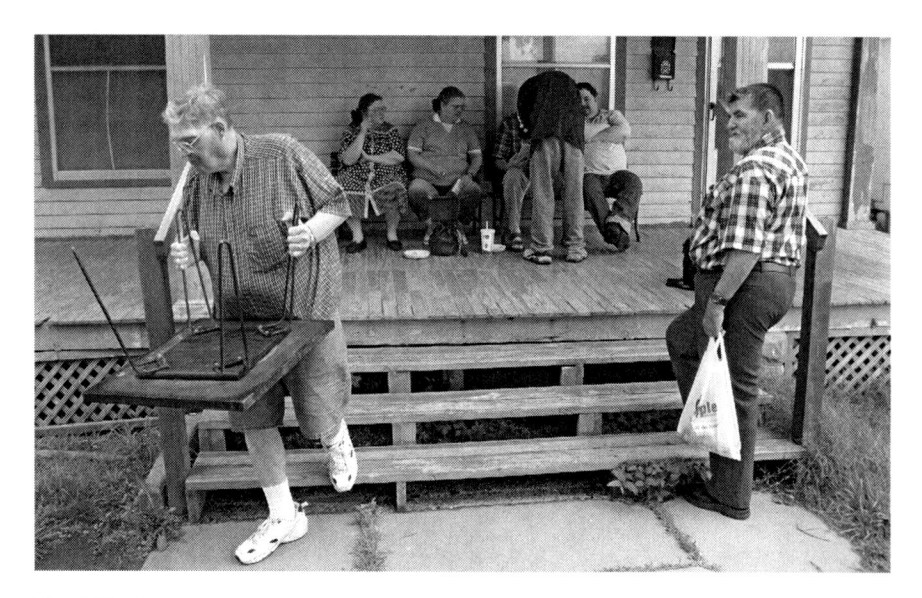

Fig. 5.37 Carl volunteered to help to move the P.S. Club furniture to their new location. After spending 11 years in the same house, the Sumner Mental Health Center decided it was time to abandon the house they were renting to the P.S. Club. They were able to provide the P.S. Club a smaller but nicer house two doors down for the same price of $300 a month

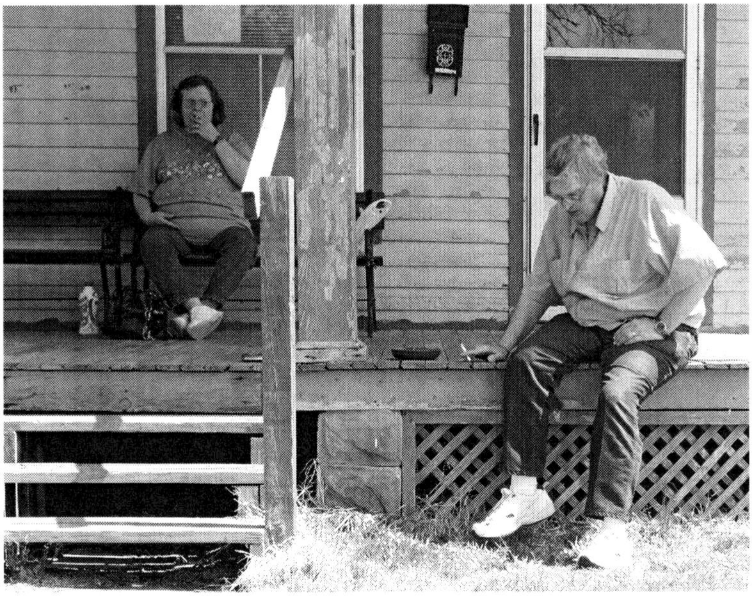

Carl's Story

Fig. 5.38 The P.S. Club and its members have different moods. Some days everyone is joking around having a good time and other days people keep to themselves

For Carl, patience and self-esteem are intertwined:

Louis: What have you done to learn to have patience?
Carl: Work on my attitude about myself.
Louis: What do you mean work on your attitude about yourself?
Carl: Well, I used to have a very low esteem of myself. I think a lot more of myself now. For instance, anybody, I don't care who they are, can think of ten things they don't like about themselves. But for each one that you write down, write down something you do like and cross out one on the list you don't like so you're not looking at that but you're looking at what you do like. And for each one you find that you write down that you like about yourself cross another one, keep crossing out as you think of things you do like and the next thing you know you got ten things you do like about yourself. Concentrate on those.
Louis: That's an interesting technique
Carl: Its helped, its helped me a lot. Because I've also used that in some peer counseling I've done. I've done a lot of peer counseling in the past 15 years. In finding ways to help me help somebody else has actually helped me too.
Louis: In what way has it helped you?
Carl: It helped me become a better person in my attitude about myself.
Louis: So it's kind of helped build your self-esteem?
Carl: Yes.

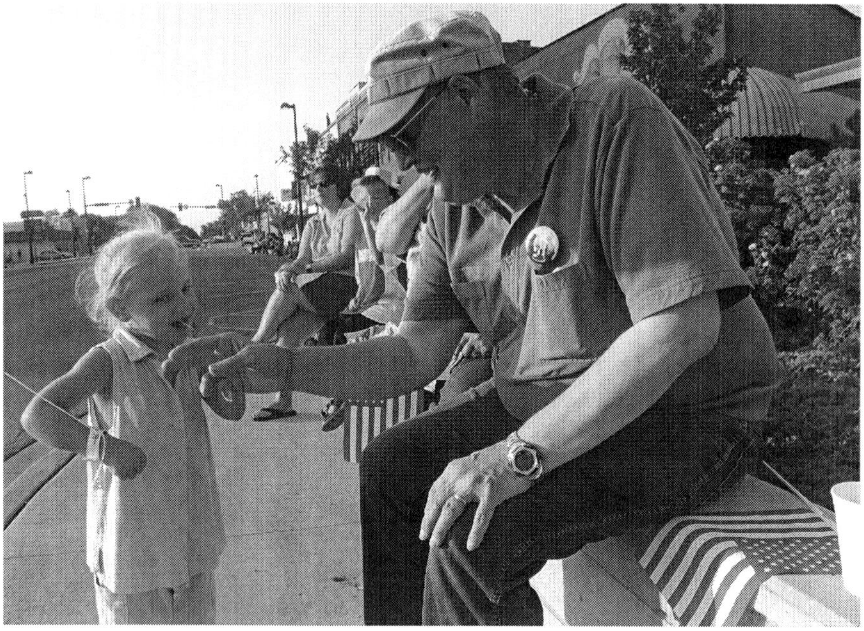

Fig. 5.39 Carl's friendly disposition is one indicator of the progress he has made towards recovery from severe depression. Pictured here, Carl enjoys interacting with a child at the Wellington Parade, which he attended with Mary

The P.S. Club has provided Carl an opportunity to help other people, which in turn has improved his self-esteem. "I never want to lose that feeling of being wanted at the P.S. Club," he says. Carl has also developed the ability to joke with others through his interactions at the P.S. Club. "It's kind of fun sometimes too, to be the brunt of a joke, to know that they can have fun with me," he says. "Cause I remember times in my life when you couldn't joke with me, I was always very serious all the time."

Although recovery is a long and arduous journey, Carl has committed himself to continue fighting. "Just because I've lost something I'm not gonna give up. I'm not gonna lay down and quit. I'm gonna keep doing things" (Fig. 5.39).

Joe's Story

"In the little town that I grew up, we were the 'niggers.' Black people weren't allowed to live there so they appointed certain [White] families to be the lowlifes. Well, my family was the lowest of the lowlifes." Growing up in the dustbowl of Kansas during the great depression, Joe's family was desperately poor. At one point he hadn't eaten for 3 days. His stomach was swollen. Out of desperation, his father stole a bag of flour from the store. His mom cooked up some biscuits quickly and everyone ate. The next day police came to his house, arrested his father, and seized the bag of flour. Joe didn't eat again for several more days.

Joe's parents came to see themselves as lowlifes and reinforced what everyone else in town communicated to Joe, that he was scum and didn't deserve anything. This message stuck and it continues to haunt Joe to this day, standing at the root of his struggles with severe depression. "In my mind, I've always been that barefoot boy with overalls on – poor White trash," he says.

Despite his impoverished upbringing, Joe had the protective factor of being bright and intellectually curious. Passionate about history, Joe read, "a series of books about yay long [stretching his arms wide] and when I was working at Cessna, I had read through that and wrote some about it." At the age of 30 he was coaxed by some of his coworkers to enroll in college. "History courses were a breeze. I'd already read all that stuff years ago."

Just when Joe started to do well, he began to feel he was not worthy of his success and sank into a deep depression. "I had a breakdown my sophomore year and I didn't drop the classes, I just quit," he says. Joe eventually came out of his depression and got both his bachelors and his masters degree by the age of 42. "Other than that [the breakdown], I would have graduated with a 4.0," he says.

After graduation, Joe started teaching high school English. Depressive episodes continued to plague him, however, forcing him to quit two jobs. "Fortunately I just had a very good friend as the head of the English department at Wichita State and when I quit [at the high school], he immediately hired me for the University so I didn't get a chance to go very deep into depression that time," he says.

The new position proved to be the best years of his life. "I was at a level that I could handle readily and I was doing a damn good job of it," he says. "So I felt good those years." Unfortunately, when Joe went up for tenure after 7 years on the job, he did not have his doctoral thesis finished and so he lost his job. Extensive research papers were never a problem, however, and what really kept Joe from receiving his doctorate was the feeling that he was not worthy of anything so honorable. "Although, it's kind of amusing, I once turned in a paper when I was working on my masters degree. Well, it was a research paper about 200 pages long and my advisors told me I should use that as a doctoral thesis but never did," he remembers.

Joe went back to teaching high school after his stint at the University. "I've never even felt comfortable in the teacher's lounge at Wichita State because I really didn't feel I belonged. As a high school teacher I was, if you pardon the expression, a star!" he says. "No, not difficult at all for me to be an outstanding teacher because I was really dedicated to it. I spent my summers preparing things for the next school year rather than taking a vacation." His success as a high school teacher continued for several years. "I love kids and I love teaching and I felt useful," he says.

Unfortunately, two rotten classes strung together ended Joe's teaching career. "I get in a situation where I don't think I can handle and I can't handle it," he says. Discipline problems shook his self-confidence. "It was all in my head," he admits.

Without anything else to do, Joe sunk into a deep depression. "I just stayed in my house and let the filth pile up. The trash on my living room floor was the size of the table. There were mice living on my dining room table," he says. Eventually the mess was reported and the Sumner Mental Health Center intervened by

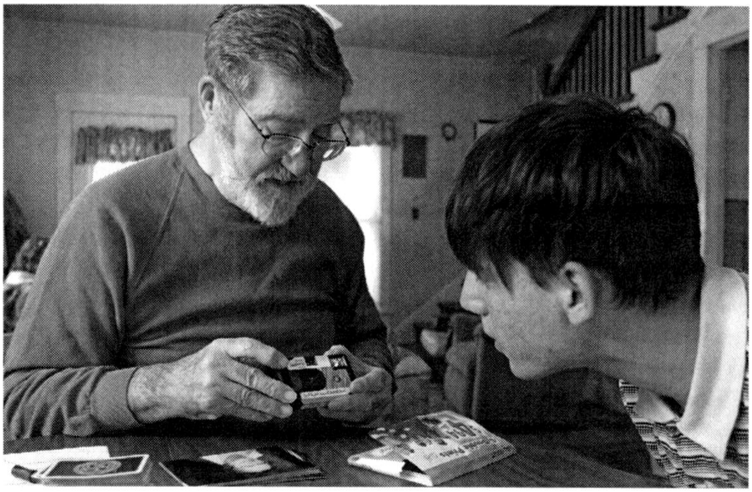

Fig. 5.40 As a part of a photovoice project at the P.S. Club, Joe fusses with the operation of a camera

sending a case manager to Joe's house. "What this case manager did that salvaged me from the trash heap was she gave me some advice that's been useful ever since, and that is, 'focus outside.' Don't focus on yourself, focus outside and that's what I've done." Although Joe's case manager has since moved away, her intervention continues to work. "I'll always be grateful to her because she straightened me up," claims Joe.

As part of focusing outside himself, Joe stated attending the P.S. Club. He was one of the original members, joining only 1 month after the Sumner Mental Health Center started the psychosocial group in 1986. Following his involvement in the P.S. Club, Joe became the consumer representative on the board of the Sumner County Mental Health Center and a volunteer at the Chisholm Trail Museum. In these positions Joe is able to be productive and contribute to society, achieving two goals he holds dear.

As a member of the P.S. Club, Joe enjoys the recreational activities. Playing cards, pool, and joking around with others are some of his favorites. "When we play cards, that's good. We're all cheerful. We all make wise remarks to each other and that's a heck of a lot of fun," he says (Figs. 5.40 and 5.41).

One activity that Joe hates is watching TV. "I can't stand that for any more than a few minutes but a good many afternoons, Mondays and Wednesdays, everybody will be sitting there, staring at the idiot box," says Joe. "It bores me to tears! Not to tears but to vacancy. I leave pretty quickly." As someone who finishes reading a book nearly every day, the TV does not typically provide Joe with enough intellectual stimulation.

Joe's intellectual nature can bring a new and welcome dynamic to the club. At times, he engages others by discussing topics such as politics and world events.

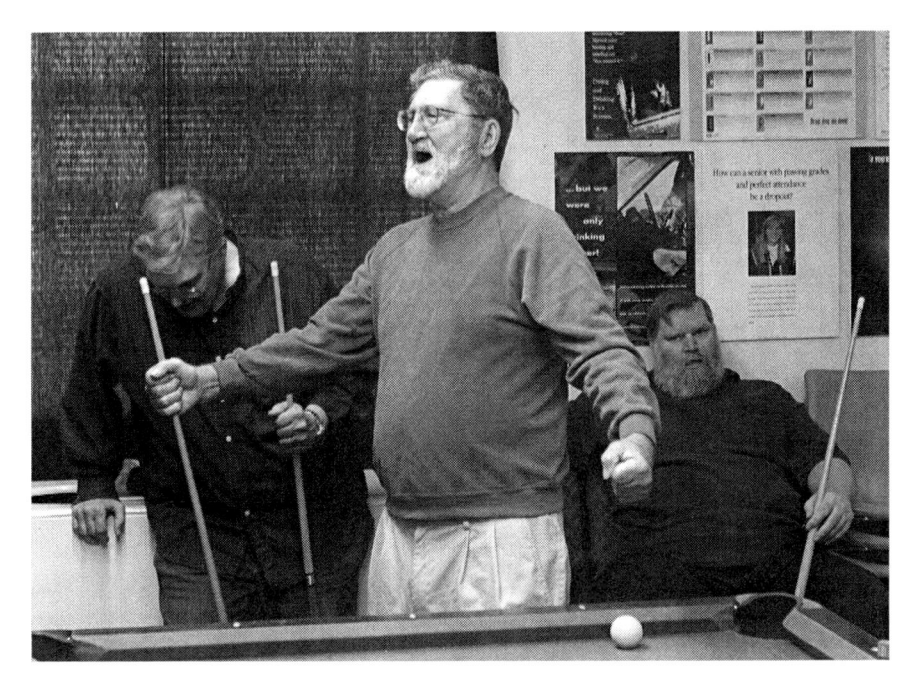

Fig. 5.41 When Joe plays pool, the balls don't always go where he wants them. He responds with playful protest

Other times his intellectual nature makes both himself and others uncomfortable. Joe's world is full of history books that others know nothing about. Trying to discuss such topics can lead to a frustratingly disjointed conversation.

Further separating Joe from other P.S. Club members is his critical and argumentative nature. "I know I am curmudgeon," he says. When he vocalizes discontent, tension in his relationships builds. Most recently, Joe has criticized the P.S. Club because its decision making is dominated by Nick. "Decisions are made for us but not by us," says Joe.

Joe wants to be more involved in the leadership of the organization. During the election for officers of the board of directors, Joe ran for president, vice president, secretary, and treasurer. He won none of these positions and was not put on the board. Joe thought the elections were unfair because Nick's family (six of the twelve people at the elections) ultimately decided who won each position, voting in two of Nick's family members as president and vice president (Fig. 5.42).

The argument led Joe towards sparse attendance. "I don't like it at all but there's nothing I can do about it except register my protest by staying away." Today Joe feels distant from everyone at the P.S. Club. "I've never gotten very close to anybody here. We're friends but in a casual sort of way," he says. Before the fight, however, Joe wrote warm descriptions of several P.S. Club members as a part of a photovoice

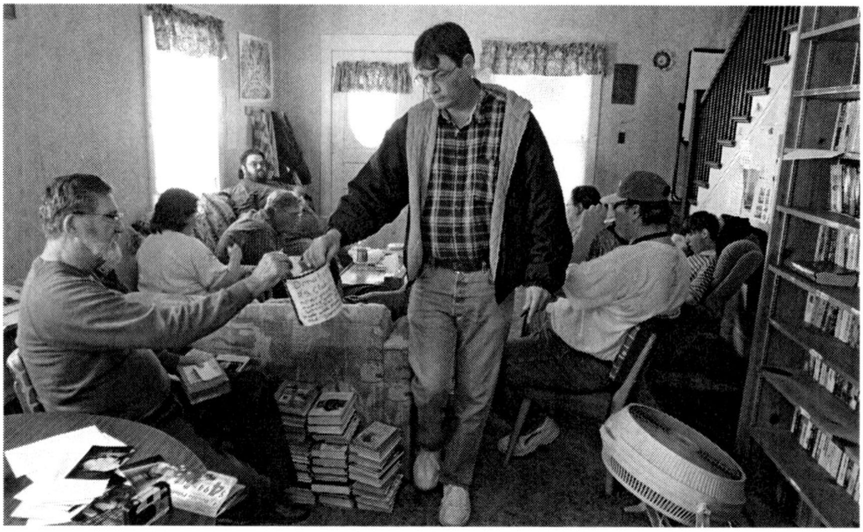

Fig. 5.42 The election of the board of directors is a yearly activity. All officer positions, including president, vice president, treasurer, and secretary must be filled by people with psychiatric diagnoses. Pictured here, Nick collects a vote from Joe for the position of secretary

project. "[Kevin] has worked his way into our affections here at the club," writes Joe. He describes another member as "a faithful, loving person and a good friend."

Without companionship, Joe is miserable. "I'm so damn lonely," he says. As an elderly man, Joe is ready to die and looks forward to oblivion. "I want to be useful and when you're no longer useful there is no point left in life." Being useful is partially what drew Joe to the club in the first place. "I've served as president of the P.S. Club and various other offices but, frankly, I don't seem to be welcome any more," he says. "I am a gadfly I guess you would say because I don't agree with a great deal that goes on around here."

In absence of the P.S. Club, Joe spends more time reading books and writing fiction in his home. More than anything else, Joe wants "to do something positive, not sit on my can and watch television." A poem, selected by Joe, about being old and useless aptly describes his current worldview (see Appendix C). "I'm just depressed about the low range of possibilities since I'm the age I am," he says. Hopefully Joe can find opportunities for engagement soon.

Kevin's Story

"All of a sudden I heard a 'MoOOoOOOo!' I look out the window, and there's the cows moving down the road. So I jumped in my four-wheeler, started it up, went and chased those cows, chased them all the way down to the gate, opened up that

Kevin's Story

gate and chased 'em into it. Then the next morning I had to go get up, just about daylight, to find out where they got out at, then go fix the fence. And so, every time I did that, they would find someplace else to break."

Such was a day in the life of Kevin for 16 years as a handyman on a farm. All of it for a room in a trailer. Disabled and living on social security income, Kevin didn't need anything else. But he loved that job because it was different every day.

Along with cows, Kevin loved trains. He would periodically take vacations across the country, riding in boxcars if he didn't have the money or Amtrak if he did. Such were the vacations of Kevin for 16 years.

Kevin remembers one trip where he went all over the country. "Went over to Chicago, from Chicago I went to New York, from New York I went to Washington DC. And on these little trips the train would stop where I could get off for a little while. I'd run around town looking for salt and pepper shakers," says Kevin. "I had this one suitcase, nothing but salt and pepper shakers."

When Kevin got back from his trip, Mrs. Jones, whom he worked for, picked him up from the train station. Kevin recalls their conversation, "she says, '[Kevin], what are you doing with that suit case?' I said, 'It's yours.' She says, 'Mine?' I said, 'YEAH! Go ahead and open it up.' She opened it up and she fell backwards! All salt and pepper shakers. She was a collector of 'em. They would fill that house up!"

Unfortunately, Mrs. Jones's daughter was not so fond of Kevin or his vacations. She had to take care of the cows while he was gone. She accused Kevin of stealing $700. He was convicted and for 13 months Kevin spent his days bored to tears in jail.

Upon release in 1995, Kevin moved to Caldwell, KS to live with his sister and help her with a paper route (Figs. 5.43–5.46). With time, Kevin moved out and his paper route ended. For $100 a month he rented a tiny, dilapidated house. For $90 a month he received hundreds of channels of satellite TV. "I just stayed here at the house, watching TV, watching TV." This was how Kevin spent his life for 7 years. Although he was in his 50s, he considered himself too old to work and was content with retirement.

In 2001, Kevin discovered the P.S. Club and quickly became the most regular of members. It became a special event if Kevin was going to miss a day. Everyone was warned ahead of time and everyone got to hear about what he did after the fact.

Nick, the executive director of the P.S. Club, drives 45 min from Wellington to Caldwell to pick Kevin up. The van rides are an opportunity for Nick and Kevin to connect. "Sometimes we talk and sometimes I'll fall asleep," says Kevin. He adds, "yeah, I'm sitting there and old [Nick] is talking to me and I'm answering him. The next thing, here I am Zzzzzzz…going like that, snoring away."

At the P.S. Club, Kevin is always ready for a game of cards. "Hey [Nick], you wanna play Phase 10 with me?" Kevin would ask on a regular basis. Skip-Bo, Phase 10, Rummy and Canasta are his favorites. Every Friday, P.S. Club members go

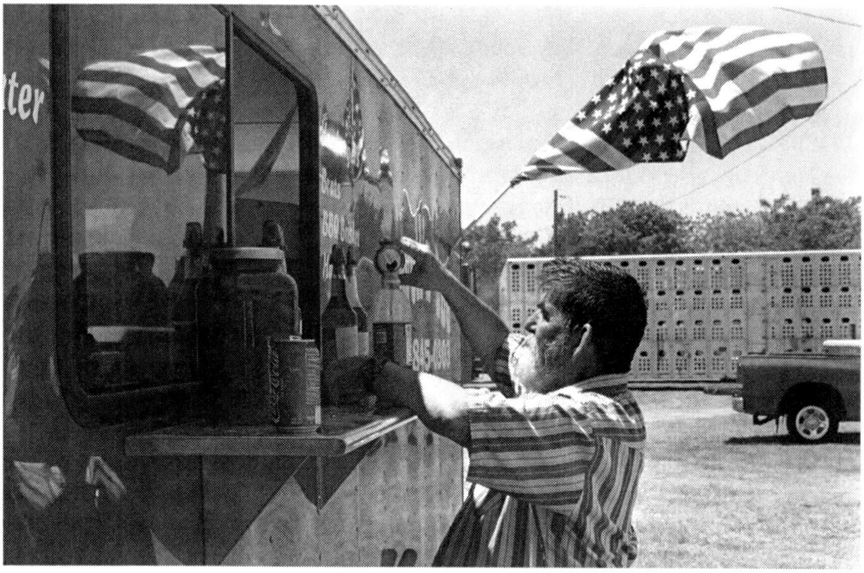

Fig. 5.43 Kevin is an avid can recycler, but he prefers to drink soda from a plastic bottle. Pictured here, he transfers soda from can to bottle at the rodeo

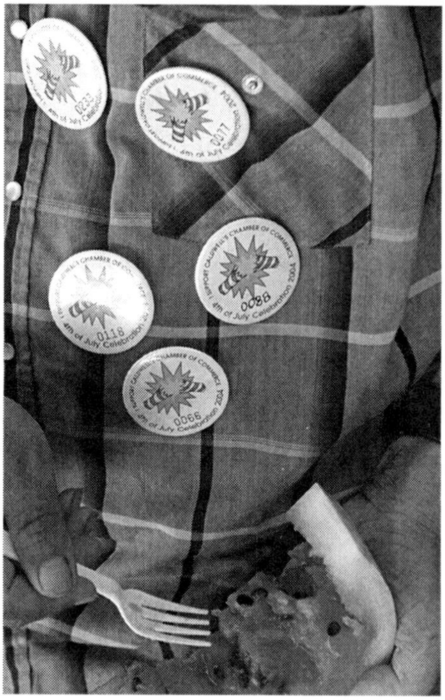

Fig. 5.44 During a Fourth of July celebration, Kevin enjoyed eating watermelon, playing bingo, and watching the fireworks. The buttons on his shirt were purchased in hopes of winning the raffle

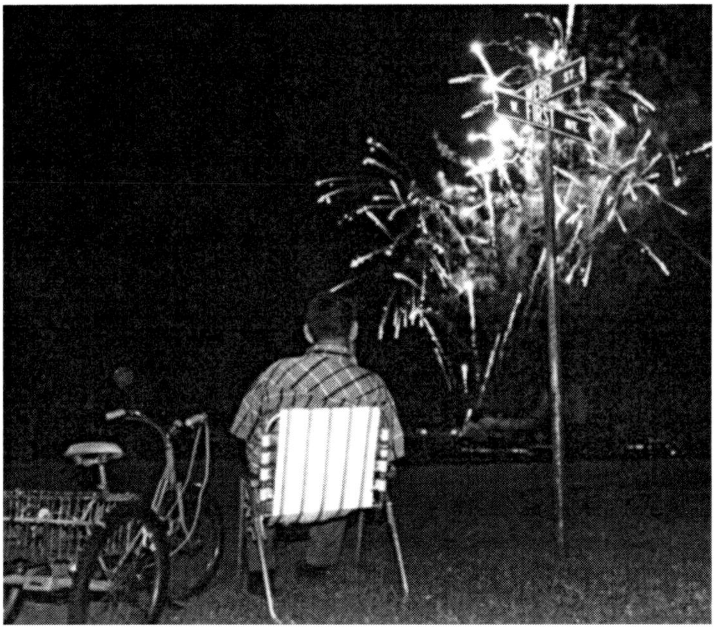

Fig. 5.45 Kevin watched the fireworks by himself. Despite living in a small, close-knit community and regularly enjoying community events, Kevin did not socialize much with others in the community

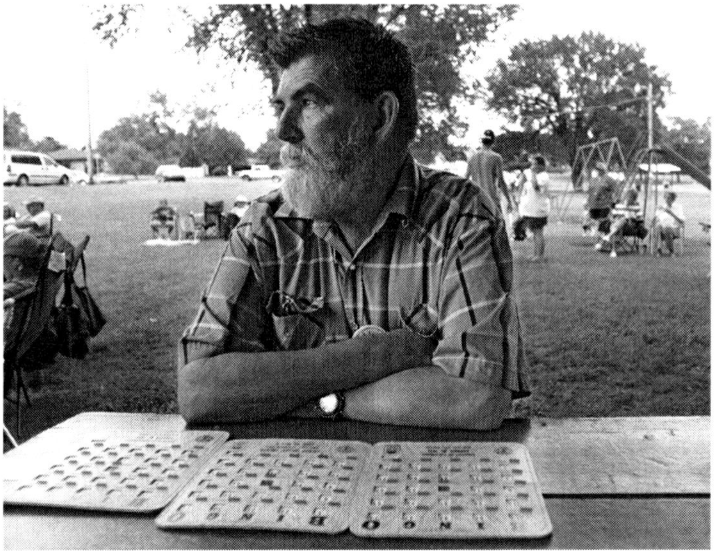

Fig. 5.46 Unfortunately, the Fourth of July was not his lucky day. None of the buttons he purchased won in the raffle and his three bingo boards produced zero wins

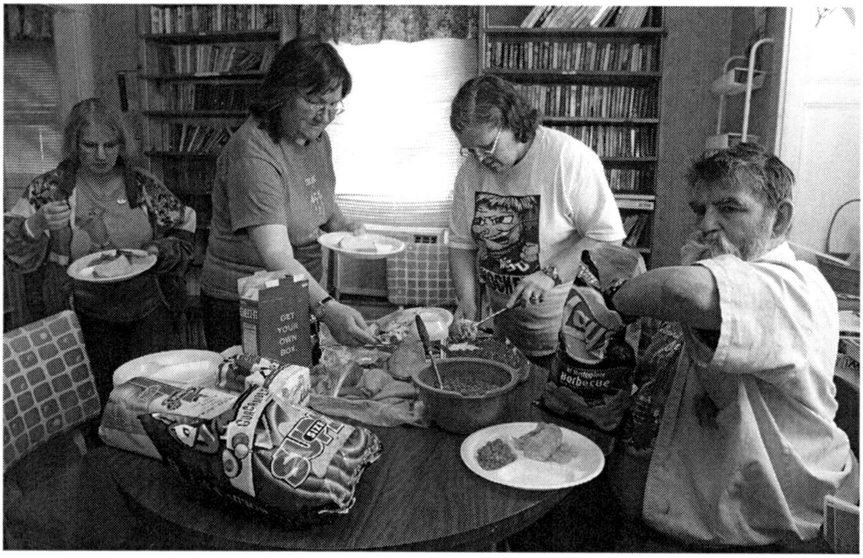

Fig. 5.47 Kevin and several other P.S. Club members enjoy a potluck lunch of ham and cheese sandwiches with baked beans, chips, and no-bake cheesecake for dessert. Potlucks are one of the more popular special events at the P.S. Club

to the Wellington Recreation Center to play pool. But pool is not Kevin's game. "No, I just want to sit on the bench. I do my crossword puzzles and watch the trains go by," he says.

Like many others at the P.S. Club, Kevin benefits from the friendships gained and the increased activity levels (Fig. 5.47). The only difference is that Kevin has never received a psychiatric diagnosis. Depression and hallucinations are foreign concepts. His dad put him on disability when he was in his twenties. "I just can't keep a job," he says, with little insight into why. While Kevin is no scholar, he is perfectly intelligent. Drugs aren't a problem either. Beer is too bitter, wine too sour, and cigarettes make him cough. At worst, he has an undiagnosed case of attention deficit hyperactivity disorder.

Although Kevin doesn't do any work at the club, he always tries to bring a smile to your face with his warm hellos and goodbyes. He shouts, "see you later alligator!," when someone leaves the P.S. Club. If you aren't coming or going, you might find yourself listening to a funny story. "This calico cat had kittens. And this one cat…this one kitten could never get in to get milk," he says. "When Blondie has her pups, that one cat came over and started sucking on Blondie. Blondie didn't care!" For Kevin, a bad experience is rare, especially at the P.S. Club. "It seems like every time I go there I have a good time," he says.

Fig. 5.48 At the 3rd Annual Chisolm Trail Bullmania, Kevin enjoyed watching the entertainment and wandering around

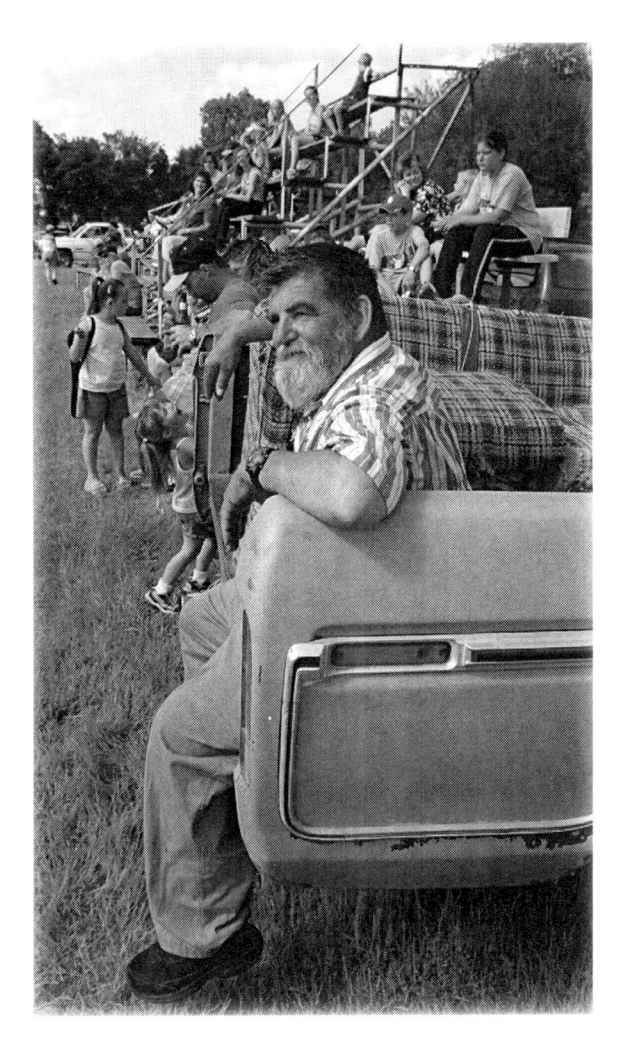

The P.S. Club never has changed his habits on the days it is closed. "Mostly, on a regular Thursday, I just stay home and watch TV, that's all that I do," he says (Figs. 5.48 and 5.49).

Epilogue – Sadly, Kevin died on February 8, 2005 at the age of 60. While the exact cause of death is unknown, his death certificate listed heart failure, respiratory problems, and high blood pressure. For someone with a disability, Kevin was remarkably healthy. He never received treatment for anything until the last year of his life. Coaxed by Nick and his sister, he went to the doctor because his hands

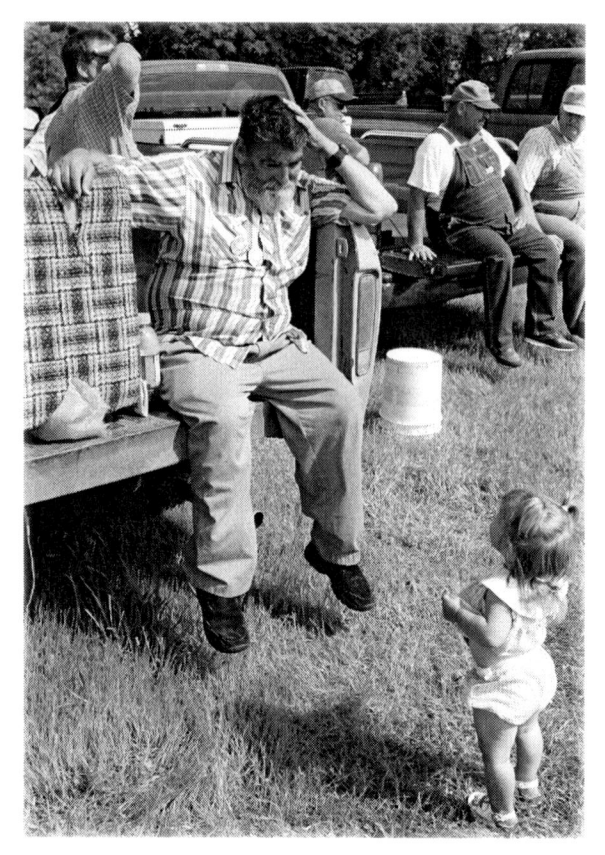

Fig. 5.49 At one point during the festival, Kevin's solitude was interrupted by a little girl who wanted to make friends

would oddly shake sometimes when he took naps. The family doctor didn't know what was wrong with Kevin and didn't make a referral for further investigation. Instead he discovered high blood pressure and gave Kevin some medication for it. A week before he died, Kevin fell out of his chair and remained unconscious when he hit the floor. Rushed to the hospital, Kevin was released hours later with no diagnosis made. Kevin died in his sleep without any medical attention.

Kevin's participation in the P.S. Club reflects what makes the organization special. It is for people with mental health problems but it is not about psychiatric diagnoses. The P.S. Club provides something basic to all humanity – a place to work, a place to play, a place to build relationships. The people who participate are the people who aren't finding these life essentials elsewhere. Kevin went because he needed social interaction just like everybody else. P.S. Club members welcomed him because they too wanted social interaction (Fig. 5.50).

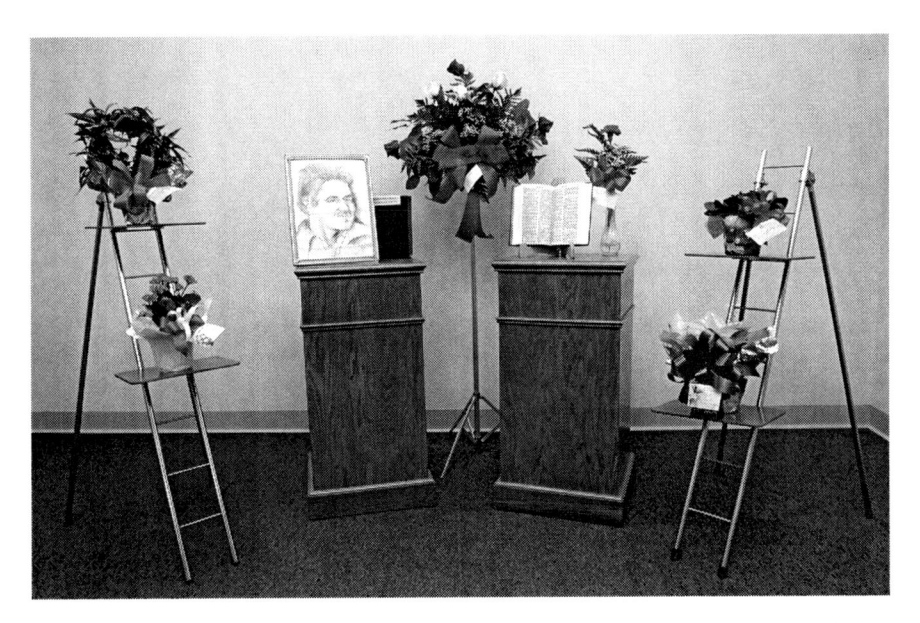

Fig. 5.50 Kevin's funeral was simple but respectfully appropriate and well attended by P.S. Club members

Laura's Story

Crummy old high school. "I'm just glad I'm out of it now," says Laura. She survived, but being teased made life miserable. Laura felt powerless against the attacks. "I knew I had to put up with it," she says.

Unfortunately, Laura's problems didn't end when she graduated from high school. "I've been trying to hold down jobs," she says. "They just didn't seem to last." Emotional problems interfered with work and her managers were never forgiving. "This one lady I knew that I was working for at this one restaurant, she didn't understand me," says Laura. "I was having these emotional times and I was getting upset because of my depression. She went ahead and fired me for no reason."

With no job and few responsibilities, life became empty. "I slept a lot and I got bored real easy," says Laura. "I got upset real easily because I couldn't find anything to do and anytime I got bored I ate." Depression became a serious problem. Medications helped her manage. "[Depression] feels like a heavy weight on you all the time and you don't feel very good about yourself but as soon as you're on the medicine it just takes that weight off."

Physical health problems with lower back pain, kidney stones, and diabetes began to complicate Laura's situation. "Mom was wanting me to live at home so she can take care of me." Medications and her family did not solve Laura's problems with boredom, however. "I complain a lot," she says. "My mom and my dad have to put up with it so they try to kind of zone me out."

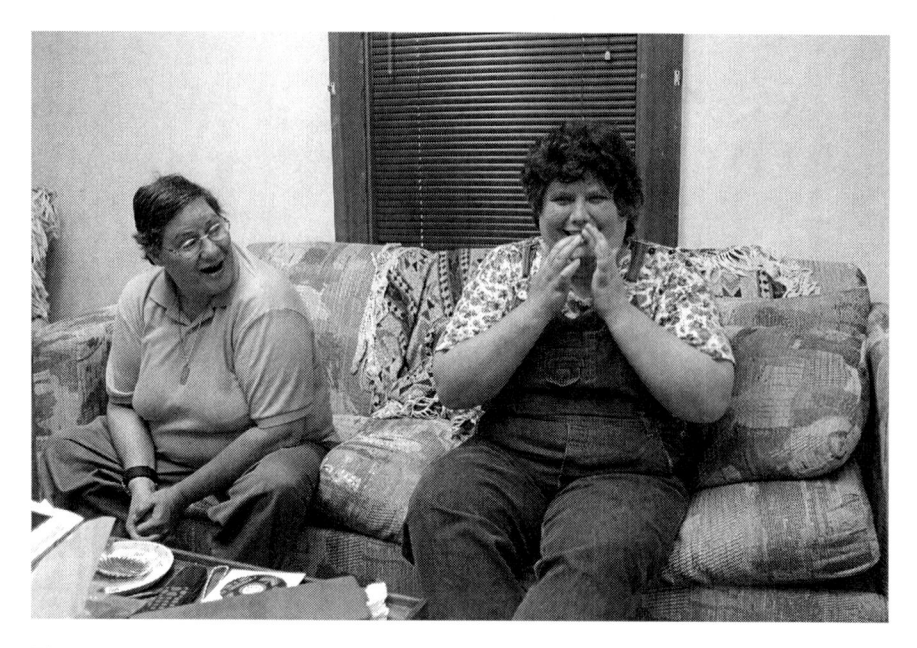

Fig. 5.51 Laura is sensitive to criticism, but when she feels accepted she is able to joke with others and enjoy herself

Laura needed friends, but friends never came easy. "My biggest challenge is to not be so shy and make friends with other people." Fortunately for Laura, she eventually met Kevin. "The first time I met him I felt like I had somebody I actually connected with," she remembers. "So me and him spent a lot of time together." It was Kevin who introduced Laura to the P.S. Club. "I didn't even know that there was club like this around for people like me," she says. "If I knew they were around sooner I probably would have joined earlier in life."

Laura saw the club as an opportunity. "I would have chances to go out and at least get away from the house for awhile and go out and make friends," she says. She enjoyed the club right from the start. "The first time I went to it I was quite excited about going to a club," she says. "I thought, well, this will be a lot of fun to go and meet new people." Laura has now been a member for 1 year and she continues to enjoy herself. "To me it's just no words to describe the P.S. Club," she says. "It's just a very good place to visit." More than anything, Laura appreciates the new social network. "Being at the club is a lot of fun you know, being around with all of your friends," she says. Laura has already generated several fond memories. "Another good experience is spending time with [Nick] and guys in the van when they are kind of laughing and picking on each other," she says. "We're just enjoying each other" (Fig. 5.51).

Laura is sensitive to criticism and the P.S. Club's warm and accepting atmosphere accommodates this sensitivity. "The people are really nice," she says. "We all seem to understand each other's feelings." At the P.S. Club Laura can be herself without fear of criticism. "There's no pressure or anything," she says. "Nobody doesn't try to step into your space where they're going to criticize you on every-

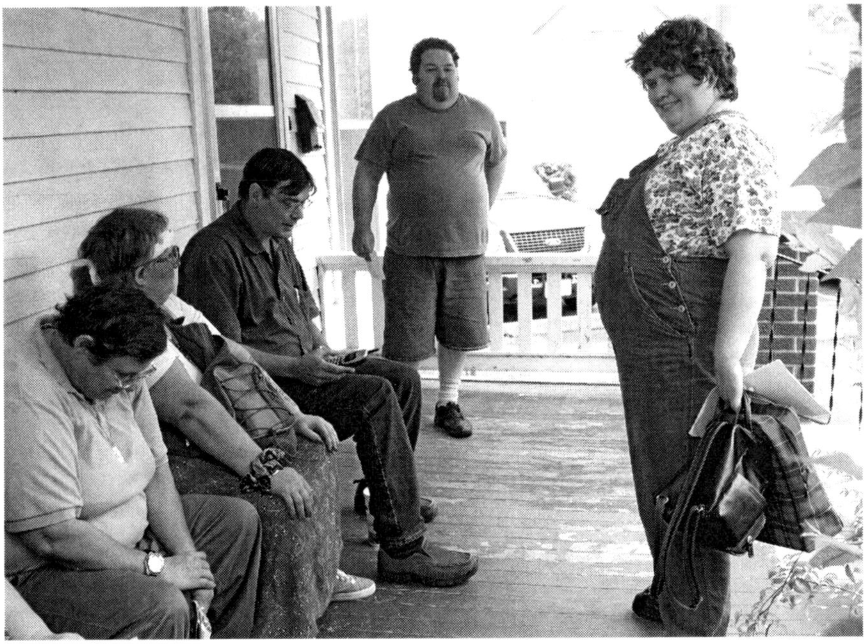

Laura's Story

Fig. 5.52 Before joining the P.S. Club, Laura struggled with boredom and loneliness. At the P.S. Club she enjoys the company of several friends and now stays more active

thing." Each member's experiential knowledge with mental health problems contributes to the pleasing atmosphere. "The person you are making friends with seems to understand the problems you are having as much as the problems they are having," she says. "They can understand how you feel."

The lives of the people Laura has gotten to know at the P.S. Club have put her own life in perspective. "You look and see other people and what they are having to go through," she says. Their stories are inspirational. "If other people can live their life through tough things I should be able to live my life through it too," she says. The power of this inspiration can be the difference between life in death during a severe depressive episode. "There are times I actually wanted to die because of the pain I was going through," she says. "With me going to this club I've been able to appreciate the life I have, even though I may go through a lot of pain."

In all of Laura's struggles, religion stands as a source of strength. "One of my strengths is being a Christian and relying on God. He is the one who guides me through all of this." Other key supports are her therapist and her family, especially her mom. "I spend a lot of time with my mom because me and my momma are really connected with each other," she says. P.S. Club members serve as a safety net of social support. "It's just like going to a second home," she says. "So far I haven't [needed help] but I believe that they probably will [help]. I really do believe that."

Laura's quality of life hinges on her continued involvement with the world. "A good day would be a day when I'm able to find things to do." The P.S. Club is now something Laura "finds to do." It's part of a good day (Fig. 5.52).

Sue's Story

As a little kid, Sue heard voices. They were her playmates. During adolescence the voices turned increasingly sour. Despite the distress, Sue maintained an "A" average in school. "I wanted so much to be the child my parents could be proud of, so I became an overachiever striving for perfection," she says. Her good grades did not equate to self-confidence in her abilities. "I use to torment my mother that way, tell her 'I think I just flunked that test, I just don't feel good about that test,'" she remembers. "Of course, she'd be concerned. I'd come up with an A+ and she was about ready to strangle me." Sue's strong academic performance continued until her senior year, when she suddenly started failing classes. She managed to graduate anyway and move on to college but it wasn't long before she was on academic probation.

For several years Sue struggled to maintain full-time employment that would pay her full-time tuition bills. Exhaustion became the norm. The anguish of waking up to face another day brought tears to her eyes.

At 25 she experienced her first hospitalization and disengaged from the world. "When my mother would visit it was so sad when she had to leave and not take me with her," she says. "I am sure we both shed tears because of this." The hospital was a miserable place, where patients and staff were pitted against each other. "One day a patient was locked in the seclusion room and the aid would not let him out to use the restroom so he urinated under the door. The urine traveled down the hall and the aid had to clean it up," she remembers. "In a sick sort of way this really made the day for us who felt powerless."

Sue left the hospital after a few months feeling just as suicidal as when she entered. She spent the next 10 years in a partial day hospital. The transition from being miserably overwhelmed to just miserable was complete. "I had no idea what I was supposed to do with my life and I was very discouraged because it seemed I had no hope," she says. Sue recounts this period in her recovery narrative:

> If you were to ask me what I felt during the worst of my mental illness I would use words such as sadness, hopelessness, frustration, helplessness, desperation and discouragement. I was quite suicidal for years and I was desperate to fix the situation but nothing relieved my symptoms. My thoughts were obsessive, overwhelming, and unbearable as they raced through my head. The voices I was hearing were persistent and ruthless. The only way to satisfy them was to obey their commands. These voices were very real and not just thoughts in my head. I would rock back and forth as if I was ready to take off like a jet.

Sue never gave up. She learned to fight her harmful behavior. "When I had a thought to harm myself by cutting, burning, or overdosing, I just repeated in my mind that that was not an option," she says. "And it worked." Her caring nature also motivated her. "My medical doctor cares very much for me, but on one occasion I had burned and I saw a tear fall from her cheek," she says. "I promised myself then that I would not hurt someone I cared a great deal about ever again."

Sue's problems with voices subsided dramatically when she started taking Clozaril in 1992. The changes allowed her to expand her horizons. No longer was she stuck taking the same social skills and good hygiene classes she had sat through so many times at the day hospital. "I could have taught them myself," she says.

Fortunately for Sue, a new nonprofit opened its doors at the same time she gained control over her symptoms. The nonprofit was Project Independence, a CRO in Wichita, KS. Sue immediately became involved in the leadership of the organization. "We worked on the by-laws to start with on my living room floor," she remembers. Project Independence got its own space before long and Sue became "the crafts lady." Every night Project Independence was open, Sue organized a craft activity. "We did everything from leather to wood," she remembers. "We had pretty good money for craft stuff."

Sue was also the president of the board of directors. She formed a close bond with Shelly, the executive director. "We had a hilarious time there when we first started going to the grocery store to get food," she remembers. "Shelly used to be so embarrassed because our cart would be heaping and she was afraid people were thinking that we were just going to go home and eat all this food."

When Shelly was sick, Sue was left in charge. "I remember one night I was having an annual meeting," she says. "We got about 60 people there and we had to put on a show for them. Go through the financial statement and go through all that stuff for the members. And I watched her walk away on her way to the hospital. I got all of this on my own shoulders. But, it went okay. We got through it."

The successes allowed Sue's self-confidence to blossom. Operating independently gave her the space she needed to build problem-solving skills. "For our survival we had to solve problems," she says. For the first time she was the one making the decisions. "Really, that's how I grew up, in a CRO. I never really thought my opinion really meant much but you know, I learned a lot from Project Independence," she says. She learned not only that her opinion mattered but that "I could come up with good ideas or that I could be responsible for other people."

While Sue enjoyed her work at Project Independence, her desire to obtain higher education never subsided. During her years at the day hospital, "I had tried and quit and tried and quit," she remembers. She was ready to try again. She started reading children's books to build up her concentration skills. "This made sense to me, and eventually, I was able to read for longer periods and more advanced material with greater retention and comprehension," she says.

In 1996, COMCARE's vocational rehabilitation program provided her with full tuition coverage, books, and travel support to attend Wichita State University. It was a dream come true and an opportunity she couldn't pass up. The school workload forced her to disengage from her craft organizing and daily attendance at Project Independence. "I know that just broke Shelly's heart but I wanted to do well in school so I had to give up." The transition was difficult but it was simply a matter of priorities for Sue. "I wanted to make straight A's the whole time so I had to," she says.

Sue persevered through 5 years of study and in 2001 she received her B.A., majoring in psychology. She continued with school and in 2003 she received her Masters in Social Work with a 4.0 grade point average. Sue's hunger for knowledge allowed her to enjoy the journey. "What I really enjoy is studying something and

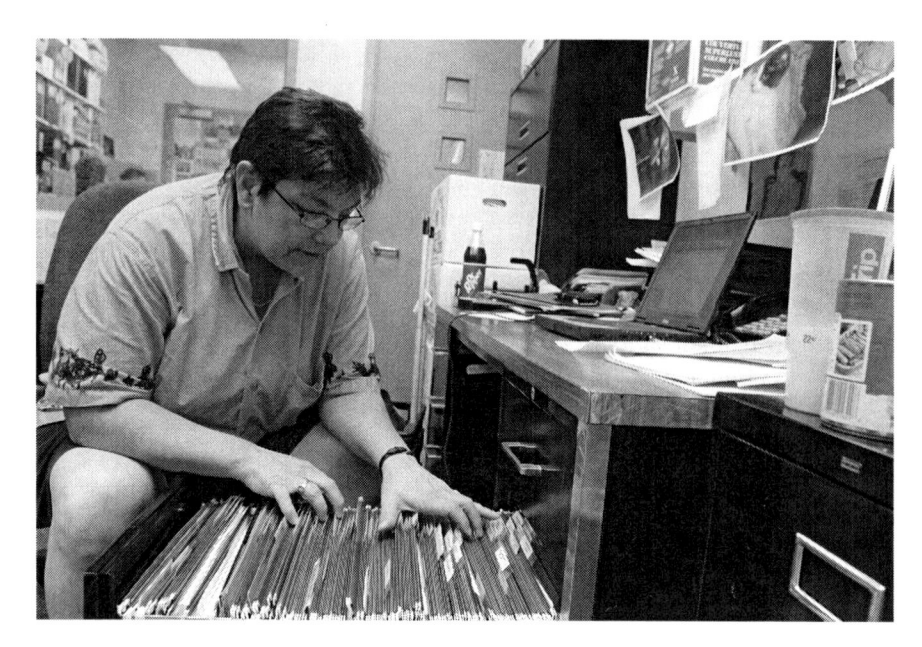

Fig. 5.53 As an employee of the Center for Community Support and Research, Sue works hard to keep her paperwork organized

then sharing the knowledge with someone. I figure if you don't share the knowledge then it's not really worth the time."

As a Master's student Sue was able to apply her knowledge during an internship with the Center for Community Support & Research. Upon graduation she was hired full time. Only 1 in 500 of the people with a mental illness on Social Security Disability Income ever get off of it. Sue is the exception to the rule the other 499 people follow. "This has been my dream since I was 25 years old and I am now 45. The math tells us that it took me 20 years to fulfill my dream, but the 'ah hah' is that I never gave up," writes Sue in her recovery narrative.

Transitioning from the role of full-time student to the role of full-time employee was a difficult one for Sue to make. "It's not uncommon for me to come home from work and just hit the couch and I'm out," she says. "Then I'm able with a good night's sleep go through it the next day." It's a tough life but Sue has no regrets. "I know that doesn't sound like much of a life but really, really it is," she says. "From doing nothing but smoking cigarettes, drinking coffee, and sitting around with people and wasting your life away to doing something productive." Independently supporting herself and helping others along the way means the world to Sue. "[I] just wanted to a do the best I could as a member of society," she says (Fig. 5.53).

Sue brings passion and a unique perspective to her work at the Center for Community Support and Research. "I feel more like I have something to contribute, that I am a part of the team and they listen to what I say," she says. "I'm not just the person that beat mental illness." She teaches a college course for people with mental

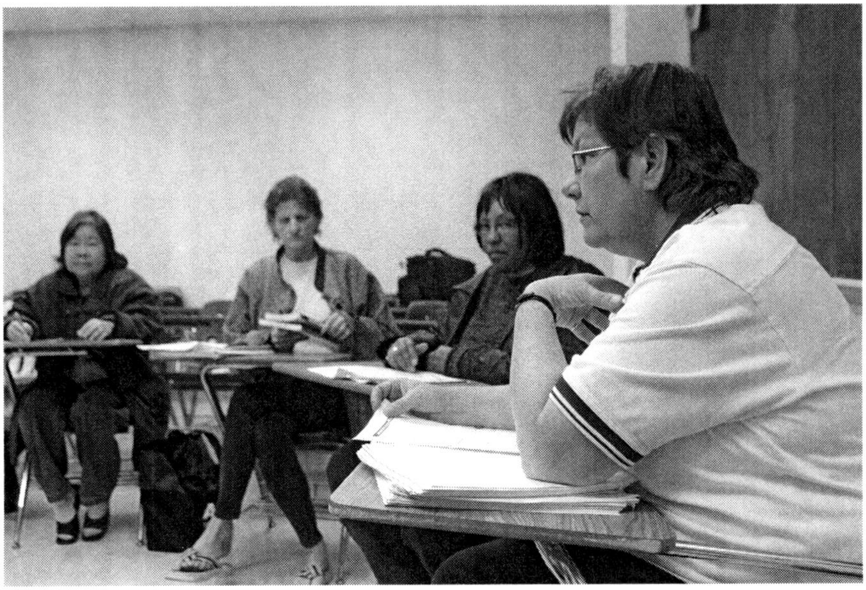

Fig. 5.54 Sue teaches the Leadership Empowerment Advocacy Project using an informal style. She sits in a desk like everyone else and facilitates group discussion

health problems called the Leadership Empowerment Advocacy Project (LEAP). "I like to give them something that they can hang on to if they are having a hard time, to make an impression on someone that's not just easily forgotten but something that changes somebody's life for the better," she says. "I think that's what makes it worth getting in front of people and speaking" (Fig. 5.54)

In addition to her teaching she provides technical assistance to CROs in Kansas. Caring Place in Newton and the P.S. Club are the two organizations she primarily supports. In all of Sue's work with CROs she is careful not be pushy. "My influence should be just to be a sounding board but not to run the show," she says. "We do have a lot of influence on our CROs. We have to be very careful not to abuse that."

In providing technical assistance to the P.S. Club, Sue helps with a variety of organizational challenges from computer problems to board training to grant writing. "I go there when everything is going great and I go there when there is a problem," she says. "I believe in relationship building." Sue especially enjoys building relationships with the P.S. Club members. "We do a lot of joking around, that's a lot of the relationship building," she says. "We always sit and have lunch together and mingle with the rest of the members." Sue's style of interaction is informal. "I got my LMSW but I don't feel like a professional," she says. "I feel more like I'm going out and I got buddies here that need some technical assistance and I try to help them with what I know." Her assistance is about more than just technical knowledge, though. "I think the main ingredient is support, some empathy and support," she says.

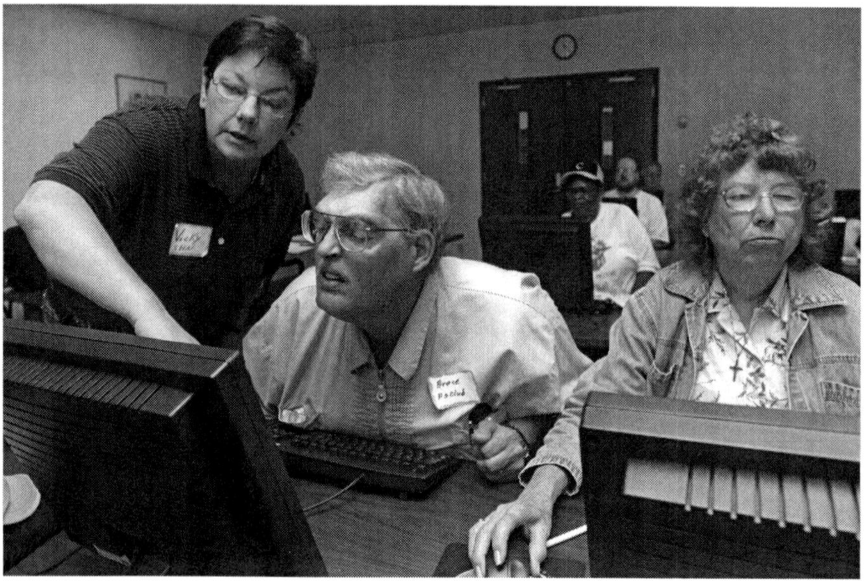

Fig. 5.55 Sue is a patient helper who never rushes the process. Pictured here Sue helps Carl learn how to use Microsoft Office applications at a computer training workshop

Sue is as much a part of the P.S. Club as the members are. "I feel like I contribute something so I feel a part of it," she says. Success for the P.S. Club is success for Sue. When schools finally started to show interest having the P.S. Club come and speak, Nick was ecstatic. "The look on [Nick's] face, you knew he was really so happy," she remembers. "After all that hard work and it just paid off. It was a good feeling I had for him." Facing problems is just as gratifying. "Being there with the problems, knowing that we can problem solve and come up with solutions. It's all very rewarding," she says (Fig. 5.55).

As someone with mental health problems who tries to help others with mental health problems, Sue tries to serve as a role model. "I have several people that look to me as a role model. They wanna get where I am today but everyone has to find their own path." Sue is especially adept at relating to and working with other people with mental health problems. "It kind of really puts a little sense into ten years in a day hospital," she says. "I'm able to use my experiences now and it wasn't all wasted years."

While Sue helps others with mental health problems she does not let them become dependent upon her. "I don't want to take the place of a therapist or take the place of a case manager. That's not the kind of role that I want. I don't want to take care of them," she says. "I want them to take care of themselves because that's the only way to make it in this world."

Despite all of the progress Sue has made towards recovery, there are still major challenges she faces every day. Her medicine doesn't work perfectly and she continues to struggle with hallucinations at times. This stress, along with her job, keeps her regularly exhausted. "The drive sure can wear you out," she says. Her ambitions have social consequences as well. "I'm just too tired to really even have a social life," she says. Success at work is more important to her. "I have a good life now and I know it's lonely at times but I just play with the cats if I get lonely," she says. Pets, including a dog, a lizard, two cats, and countless fish welcome her every time she comes home. "I ought to just live in a zoo," she jokes.

Sue's accomplishments bring her pride but she is not about to rest on her laurels. "I'd like to finish my Ph.D. and write a book," she says. For now however, Sue is staying put. "I'm content where I'm at," she says. "I still have the drive to go even farther but for right now I'm okay."

Chapter 6
Using Narratives to Understand How People Benefit from CROs

Abstract In this chapter, I analyze the life history narratives of consumer-run organization (CRO) participants from an etic or outsiders' perspective using the role framework as a guide. Each narrative is individually analyzed with an emphasis placed on how the narratives can and cannot be understood using the role framework. The analyses conceptually organize each life history into the components of the role framework. The resulting write-up for each key informant provides insight into the utility of the role framework. The analyses also improve conceptual understanding of how each informant's life changed over time, along with how each participant did and did not benefit from CRO participation. After the individual analyses, the chapter provides an integrative summary analysis of all narratives.

This chapter explores how the life histories can be explained using the role framework. Theoretical analysis occurs first with each individual life history. Following the individual analyses is a summary and conclusion section that individually addresses each component of the role framework. Stage-specific confirming and disconfirming evidence from all of the life histories is reviewed. Following each review, conclusions are made on the usefulness of each stage in understanding how people benefit from CRO participation.

Theoretical Analysis of Mary

Component One: Person–Environment Interaction

The P.S. Club provides Mary an accepting environment where people exercise patience when she struggles with cognitive difficulties. The P.S. Club also provides a unique work environment where she can thrive when she is feeling well. If she is feeling overwhelmed, she can take the day off without fearing repercussions. If she is hospitalized, her job is still waiting for her when she gets out.

Component Two: Role and Relationship Development

Outside of the P.S. Club, Mary plays the role of dependent mental health client. Inside the club, Mary developed both friendship and leadership roles. She has close friendships with several members. These relationships are particularly important because she does not have close friends outside of the club. Her only leadership roles are with the club, where she works as a shift manager and as treasurer of the board of directors.

Although she is glad to have her work and friendship roles, they do have downsides. All of them can bring her unwanted stress that increases her anxiety. Mary struggles to strike a delicate balance between boredom and overload. Not doing enough allows her to dwell on her paranoia and anxiety, making them worse. Doing too much can overwhelm her, increasing her anxiety. Her job is sometimes more than she can handle. Fortunately Mary can get someone to fill in for her if she is not feeling well. Although Mary's friends at the P.S. Club are also generally helpful, some people are a source of stress for Mary. Like the psychiatric clients whom Estroff (1985) studied, Mary prefers the social code, "keep your crazies to yourself" (p. 63). The abnormal behavior of others can be distressing.

Component Three: Resource Exchange

In her friendship and leadership roles, Mary finds interdependence in co-equal supportive relationships. In her employee role she helps the organization stay organized and clean. The small paycheck also provides her with needed tangible resource support, helping her make it to the next social security check.

In her role as friend she both helps and is helped by her friends. Sharing her struggles with others helps her to digest and understand them. She always listens attentively when others need to share their own struggles. In this listening exchange, a mutual appreciation develops. Mary also likes to joke with people and tell funny stories when she can.

Component Four: Self-Appraisal

Mary's friendships at the P.S. Club help her feel valued. She is always good natured and people at the P.S. Club like her. She knows this and she feels comfortable there. All of these supportive exchanges make her feel good about herself.

Mary is also trusted with the responsibility of being the treasurer, which helps promote her self-esteem. She takes pride in this prestigious position, as it reflects her competence as an individual. The job helps her combat feelings of inadequacy and ineptitude.

Component Five: Building Role Skills

Mary does not readily identify skills which she developed through CRO participation. It may be that she already possesses the skills necessary to successfully meet her role expectations at the P.S. Club.

Component Six: Identity Transformation

Mary's friendships and job at the P.S. Club provide her with a sense of normalcy despite her struggles with mental health problems. She wants to identify as a normal person and live a normal life. Her identification with her "normal" roles helps to inspire her to keep fighting the demons of her mental health problems.

Although Mary's life at the P.S. Club gives her hope, she still identifies as someone who is very dependent on the help of others. Without her case manager, her attendant care worker, and her doctor, she would be lost. She serves as an example of the limits of CRO participation. The cognitive difficulties caused by schizophrenia simply cannot be adequately addressed or resolved through CRO participation alone. Mary is, however, more involved in life, and her participation is an important source of self-esteem, psychological well-being, and tangible resource support.

Theoretical Analysis of Nick

Component One: Person–Environment Interaction

The P.S. Club provided Nick with a working environment where he could thrive. Whenever he felt stressed, he was able to take a break rather than pushing ahead in the face of worsening psychiatric symptoms. The club also provided an atmosphere where he felt comfortable making friends. The recreational activities offered by the club served as a medium through which friendships developed.

Component Two: Role and Relationship Development

Nick developed many close friendship roles through his participation in recreational activities at the P.S. Club. In his leadership role as director, he filled a variety of helper roles, such as transportation provider, grant writer, accountant, public speaker, and staff manager. These new roles gave Nick's life a purpose. Nick also evolved out of dependency roles during his involvement in the P.S. Club. His former therapist became a colleague who works in the mental health system. His only reliance on the professional mental health system became a need for medication. Nick also stopped relying on his parents for material support.

Component Three: Resource Exchange

Although this was not always the case, Nick began to give far more in helper roles than he received in dependency roles. As a CRO member, he gave people someone to play games with, someone to share stories with, and someone who understands. His friends at the P.S. Club returned the favor. Being able to maintain gratifying friendships and recreational experiences allowed him to relieve stress and have fun, thereby improving life satisfaction. The stress relief, in turn, helped him manage his psychotic symptoms.

Component Four: Self-Appraisal

Nick obtained many positive appraisals in his friendship roles. When Nick told a joke or a funny story and everyone laughed, he wasn't just exchanging chuckles. The underlying message embedded in those laughs was that people enjoyed Nick's company. The positive appraisal was reflected back to Nick, which led to a positive self-evaluation. His self-esteem increased. Nick became wanted and needed because he brought people joy.

Of course, one good joke will not change a life, but a habit of joking can. Nick's sense of humor was valued at the club. He brought a life to the club that was often absent without his presence. As a result, everyone at the club loved Nick. Rather than communicating their feelings about Nick with words, they frequently used laughter. Either way, Nick got the message, and it made him feel good about himself.

Component Five: Building Role Skills

In his role as director, Nick learned many skills, especially public speaking and accounting skills. Nick did not, however, attribute his reduction in shyness to his participation in the P.S. Club. Instead, his psychiatric medication reduced his paranoia, enabling him to communicate comfortably with non-consumers who do not understand mental health problems. Social interaction was no longer a frightening experience. When the paranoia lifted, dormant social skills emerged, and Nick became able to socialize with ease.

This shows that simply maintaining roles and relationships does not automatically lead to skill development. Nick socialized at the P.S. Club for years without seeing an improvement in his social skills or his ability to adeptly socialize elsewhere. The P.S. Club provided a uniquely understanding and accepting setting where Nick was comfortable socializing. He was not only comfortable but good at it. Nick was able to use his existing social skills at the P.S. Club effectively. He simply needed a reduction in fear of the other social situations in order for his social skills to emerge in other settings.

Component Six: Identity Transformation

Nick's reluctance to initially join the P.S. Club was due in part to his lack of identification as someone with a severe mental health problems. Diagnosed only two years earlier, he was still hoping doctors had made a mistake. Participation in the club required him to accept his identity as someone with a mental health problems. However, it also provided him opportunities to develop helper roles, where he could defy the expectations of incompetence associated with receiving a psychiatric diagnosis. Through his P.S. Club involvement, he stopped being ashamed of his psychiatric diagnosis and started being able to share his experiences openly with large groups of strangers. Instead of accepting the limited expectations associated with his diagnosis, he committed himself to fighting the stigma through his public presentations. He began to see himself as a leader, serving as a role model for others at the P.S. Club. He also began to see himself as more independent because he has transitioned out of dependency roles with his parents and his therapist.

Theoretical Analysis of Carl

Component One: Person–Environment Interaction

At the Club, Carl found a friendly, understanding, and encouraging environment that provided him opportunities to make friends and become involved in organizational leadership. This helped him to address personal problems at the root of his depression, including loneliness, low self-worth, and an inadequate sense of competence.

Component Two: Role and Relationship Development

Carl played several roles at the P.S. Club, including that of friend, peer counseling coordinator, shift manager, and board member. These new roles and relationships helped Carl address problems with loneliness, which stood at the root of his depression.

Component Three: Resource Exchange

Playing the role of friend at the P.S. Club provided Carl with opportunities to exchange laughter, social support, empathy, advice, and intimate personal information. In his organizational roles, he received some financial compensation for his efforts to support the P.S. Club. He also received gratitude from many people for his efforts.

Component Four: Self-Appraisal

The organizational leadership roles provided Carl with a much-needed sense of importance. He knows people want him to be involved and he uses that knowledge to ward off his tendencies toward feelings of worthlessness. Through organizational contribution, he makes himself useful and wanted, receiving positive appraisals.

His friendships and kidding with others also led to positively reflected appraisals, because people enjoyed his company and wanted to spend time with him. Carl benefits from the sense of importance he gains by knowing people in the community, and he feels good about himself when he can make others laugh. The positive appraisals from his friendship and leadership roles provide him with an important boost in self-esteem, which was immensely helpful because his childhood left him feeling worthless.

Component Five: Building Role Skills

Through his friendship roles, Carl's social skills and social confidence improved substantially. He became adept at joking with others. His ability to kid others and exchange pleasantries enabled his attainment of the positive reflected appraisals he never received as a child.

Component Six: Identity Transformation

An important identity change has occurred within Carl. He now sees himself as a fun and sociable person. His newfound identity motivated him to stay involved and active in his community. With his new identity, he not only learned to manage existing relationships but also began to seek out friendly social interaction with other residents of Wellington, KS.

Theoretical Analysis of Joe

Component One: Person–Environment Interaction

Joe deeply valued contribution to society and felt life was pointless without such involvement. At one point in time, the P.S. Club provided Joe with opportunities to get involved in leadership activities and contribute to its organizational success. Joe was also lonely and the P.S. Club was a place where he could make friends. Although he tried to interact with others in the P.S. Club environment, his personality repeatedly clashed with others at the club and with the club environment itself. He needed a highly active and intellectually stimulating setting, whereas other members preferred a slower pace and had different interests.

Component Two: Role and Relationship Development

Joe developed both friendship and leadership roles at the P.S. Club. When the roles were going well he enjoyed them thoroughly. The relationships helped him keep his focus outside of himself and away from depressing thoughts. He had a hard time maintaining his leadership roles because disagreements would lead to either conflict or disengagement on his part. His friendships at the P.S. Club were equally tenuous. He enjoyed joking with people but often had a hard time finding shared interests.

Joe's experiences at the P.S. Club are an example of the participant who gets involved, develops new roles and relationships, benefits from those relationships, but then for one reason or another, disengages from the organization, unable to replace lost roles and relationships. Unfortunately, many CRO participants experience similar patterns. Conflicts frequently arise in relationships of all kinds, including those at CROs. They make all parties uncomfortable. Without resolution, conflict continues to strain relationships, leading people toward disengagement. Conflict management and resolution skills are critical in the maintenance of roles and relationships within CROs.

Component Three: Resource Exchange

During recreational activities, Joe was successful in his friendship roles at the P.S. Club. Games sufficiently engaged his attention, allowing him to relax, exchange supportive words, kid with others, and share interesting stories in between turns. Without the recreational activities, he had a hard time connecting with members through conversation alone. He would become bored and leave because watching TV with other members did not appeal to him. When he lost his friendships at the P.S. Club, there were no resource exchanges and he became very lonely.

Component Four: Self-Appraisal

Joe's self-appraisals were persistently negative because he learned to think of himself as a lowlife during his childhood, where he was treated as a second-class citizen. Finding roles where he was able to productively contribute to society substantially improved his self-appraisals and he began to consider himself a valuable individual. For a limited amount of time, Joe was able to maintain leadership roles at the P.S. Club that enhanced his self-appraisals because he was able to contribute. Unfortunately, Joe was unable to maintain his leadership role; once it was lost, his self-appraisals declined.

Component Five: Building Role Skills

Joe did not develop new skills through his involvement in the P.S. Club. His lack of interpersonal conflict resolution skills led to multiple uncomfortable confrontations with P.S. Club members and a bad reputation. Having learned little, his life reverted to the way it was before he became involved.

Component Six: Identity Transformation

Joe struggled with his identity as "poor White trash" throughout his adulthood. Although he wanted very much to be a productive member of society, success also scared him. His sense of inferiority led him to sabotage his opportunity to become a tenured professor. However, fear of success did not prevent his involvement in the P.S. Club. Rather, it was his lack of interpersonal skills in dealing with disagreements.

Joe's situation is congruent with identity theory in that when he had no roles or relationships, he was miserable. When he did have roles and relationships, he was happier and had a stronger sense of purpose in life. As someone who maintained roles and relationships at the P.S. Club but never changed his identity or skills, Joe was left with nothing when he disengaged. Quality of life went up while he participated but it went right back to original levels when he disengaged.

Theoretical Analysis of Kevin

Component One: Person–Environment Interaction

The P.S. Club provided Kevin a welcoming opportunity to get involved in recreational activities. As an underpopulated setting, Kevin's presence was frequently needed for card and board games that required three or four willing participants.

The P.S. Club also provided an environment that did not judge him for frequently choosing to fall asleep rather than socialize when recreational activities were not underway.

Component Two: Role and Relationship Development

Kevin took full advantage of the opportunity to participate in P.S. Club activities. He was the most consistent attendee. He was always friendly and ready for a game of cards but he rarely engaged in extensive conversation. Everybody liked Kevin but he was not particularly close with anyone. When card games were not being played, he would typically watch TV or fall asleep. He was never interested in taking on leadership roles, despite having opportunities to do so. His role and relationship development replaced time otherwise spent at home alone with the TV.

Component Three: Resource Exchange

Kevin was a resource to the P.S. Club as a reliable and pleasant participant in card and board games. Everybody, including Kevin, received gratifying recreation during those games. Kevin was also a reliable resource as someone who wanted to spend time with people and enjoyed lighthearted interaction. He regularly shared stories with others and kept people up to date about events he was looking forward to, but rarely exchanged the deep intimacies of a close friend.

Component Four: Self-Appraisal

Kevin saw his working days as over. He identified as someone who was "retired," although he was in his late 50s. As such, his self-expectations were to spend his time in recreation. The P.S. Club provided him an opportunity to verify his identity. Through P.S. Club participation, he was able to engage with the world in a satisfying manner. No other place in the community was so accepting.

Component Five: Building Role Skills

Kevin did not build role skills through his participation in the P.S. Club. Personal growth and self-actualization were not his goals. He simply wanted to enjoy the remaining years of his life.

Component Six: Identity Transformation

Kevin's identity did not change as a result of CRO participation. Instead, he was better able to live his ideal life through CRO participation. Despite several opportunities and a reasonable amount of encouragement without pressure, he never expressed interest in taking on leadership roles. It simply was not an identity that he was interested to embrace.

Theoretical Analysis of Laura

Component One: Person–Environment Interaction

Prior to meeting Kevin and learning about the P.S. Club, Laura spent her time at home with nothing to do. Her social network did not extend past her mom and dad, whom she lived with. The P.S. Club provided Laura with opportunities to get involved in recreational activities and make friends in an understanding and accepting environment. The non-judgmental nature of the P.S. Club was critical to engaging Laura because of her sensitivity to criticism.

Component Two: Role and Relationship Development

The P.S. Club fulfilled Laura's combined need for recreation and a non-judgmental atmosphere. She developed new roles and relationships which have facilitated tremendous change in her life. Laura gained the role of friend, member, and activity participant. As someone who was bored at home all the time, Laura's newfound engagement was a life-changing experience. She sleeps less, complains less about being bored, and is less inclined to eat because of boredom. This more active lifestyle may lead to improvements in her physical health problems with diabetes and lower back pain.

Component Three: Resource Exchange

Laura's roles in the P.S. Club lead her to expend energy on gratifying recreation, receiving entertainment in exchange for her efforts. Everybody laughs, everybody jokes, and it feels good to be together. In her role as friend she has received important social comparison information. She has learned how much people with mental health problems can go through and how much they can overcome.

Component Four: Self-Appraisal

The warm and accepting atmosphere of the P.S. Club is sensitive to the negative reflected appraisals that Laura hates so much. Nobody criticizes her, the way kids in high school did. Replacing the negative reflected appraisals is a positive one; she and everyone around her enjoy spending time together. Through her friendship roles, Laura learned important self-relevant information about the coping power of others with mental health problems. Inspired by this information, she began to appraise her life as more valuable and see more hope for the future.

Components Five and Six: Building Role Skills and Identity Transformation

As a relatively new member who regularly attends but is not involved in any leadership roles, Laura's identity and skills have not changed substantially. It is unclear why her newfound friendship roles did not alter her skills or identity, but it may be she already possessed the necessary skills to maintain friendships, once she was provided a non-judgmental atmosphere where people could relate to her problems with depression. Her identity as a friendly person receives confirmation through her P.S. Club involvement, but involvement itself may not have required identity transformation.

Theoretical Analysis of Sue

Component One: Person–Environment Interaction

In her journey through life, Sue has seen tremendous changes in roles, relationships, skills, and identity. The thread of consistency is her ambition, a defining feature of her personality that influenced many interactions with her environment. Her psychiatric symptoms made her ambition worthless as she simply could not figure out a way to manage them enough to be a productive citizen. This frustrating circumstance caused much of her depression.

When the Project Independence CRO began to form, it provided Sue with an opportunity for her to apply her ambition to contribute to society. Although Sue jumped at the opportunity, it was not an opportunity she had the capacity to undertake while she was attending a day hospital. Second-generation psychiatric medication reduced her symptoms to the point where she was capable of getting involved in a leadership role at Project Independence.

Similarly, when Sue learned about the scholarship funding provided by COMCARE's vocational rehabilitation program, she again jumped at the opportunity because she loves learning and wanted to get the training necessary to develop an ambitious career. Although her commitment to education initially pulled her away from CROs, it eventually brought her back in her job at the Center for Community Support & Research. She was well-qualified for the job because of her previous experiences at Project Independence and her Masters in Social Work. Although she finds the work extremely demanding, she persists because of her ambition.

Component Two: Role and Relationship Development

Sue was the only person interviewed who made role transitions out of the CRO. Sue transitioned through several roles and relationships as she progressed from her role as hospitalized mental patient to one of independent, self-supporting citizen. Her first role transition was from mental patient to volunteer leader at Project Independence. Next she transitioned to the role of full-time student, eventually earning her Masters in Social Work. Then she obtained a full-time job at the Center for Community Support & Research, where she started providing other CROs such as the P.S. Club with technical assistance. Sue fully engaged herself in each role, striving not only for success but excellence. Each role served as a stepping stone, where she was able to build the skills necessary to succeed in the next phase of her life.

Component Three: Resource Exchange

At Project Independence, Sue donated significant amounts of time to her role as president of the board of directors and as crafts organizer. For Sue, the rewards were learning and personal growth. Sue was less cognizant of rewards stemming from increased social approval or a feeling of being needed. Sue deeply enjoyed the close personal friendship she forged with the director. They exchanged social support and laughter regularly. She experienced substantial loss when she left Project Independence, but the knowledge resources gained from her role as student outweighed the loss. She poured all her energy into her studies, receiving a 4.0 GPA. Her success helped her obtain a full-time job, where she uses what she learned to help others. In return, she receives enough compensation to live a comfortable and healthy middle class lifestyle.

Component Four: Self-Appraisal

Sue's involvement in Project Independence altered her self-appraisals substantially. Her successes as president of the board of directors and as crafts leader gave her self-confidence in her ability to act independently and successfully solve problems. She received positive appraisals from those who appreciated her efforts and reliably friendly demeanor, especially the director. Sue values contribution to society tremendously and her ability to contribute to the success of Project Independence substantially improved her self-confidence and self-worth. It is hard to overestimate the importance of this transformation in allowing her to succeed in her subsequent roles as student and then full-time employee. Self-confidence was a particularly imposing barrier to her entire life, irrespective of mental health problems.

Although later roles did not provide Sue with more positive appraisals, she did come to view herself more favorably. She deeply values contribution to society as a self-supporting citizen and her full-time job allows her to live in a manner consistent with her values. These internalized values are a far more powerful motivating force in Sue's life than the appraisals of others.

Component Five: Building Role Skills

In all of Sue's new roles, she developed important skills. These skills carried over to new contexts when Sue made role transitions. Although her new roles always demanded new skills, they also demanded the skills she developed in the previous roles. Her path from Project Independence to student and to employee is part of an upward spiral developmental trajectory. The importance of the improved problem-solving skills and confidence with which Sue left Project Independence cannot be overestimated. They were instrumental in helping her get through school and obtain full-time employment. Sue continues to grow and, as long as she can manage her mental health problems, her career will continue to progress. As a student, Sue developed skills in reading and writing. At her job she developed public speaking skills. She serves as a role model to many and she has come to enjoy speaking in front of large groups.

Component Six: Identity Transformation

Sue's identity has transformed along with her new roles. She sees herself as a leader whose voice is valued. She also views herself as a helpful individual who is capable of building strong rapport and effectively sharing what she has learned with others. In all of her post-day-hospital roles, she has operated independently but she was dependent upon financial support from the government. Finally, as a full-time employee, she is a financially independent, self-supporting citizen who gives back to the community, an identity she values tremendously.

Summary Cross-Case Analysis of Life History Narratives

The individual stories of P.S. Club participants provide a generally congruent body of support for the role framework. However, many people only experienced certain outcomes described by the role framework. The varied and voluntary nature of CRO participation leads people to change in different ways.

Although different people have different CRO participation experiences, leading to different outcomes, the role framework does appear to be useful in conceptualizing how these changes take place. Following is a summary of how the seven intensely studied lives can and cannot be understood using the role framework.

Component One: Person–Environment Interaction

All seven informants were socially isolated when they began interacting with the P.S. Club. The friendly, accepting, and home-like atmosphere helped informants feel comfortable. The club also organizes a variety of recreational activities that serve as a medium through which friendships develop. These characteristics were vital in keeping informants engaged, as all faced difficulties connecting with others.

The P.S. Club also provided a working environment where people with mental health problems could thrive. If Nick felt stressed, he was able to take a break rather than pushing ahead in the face of worsening psychiatric symptoms. Similarly, if Mary was hospitalized, her job was always waiting for her when she got back. Having one person fill in for another is a common and accepted practice at the P.S. Club.

Component Two: Role and Relationship Development

All life histories reflected the development of friendship roles at the P.S. Club. By forming friendships, informants transitioned from idle solitude to active engagement. This involvement prevented problems with boredom for Laura and Kevin and problems with rumination on troublesome thoughts for Mary, Joe, and Carl.

Nick, Mary, Sue, and Carl also maintained paid leadership roles at the P.S. Club. At times, Joe also maintained leadership roles at the P.S. Club. However, his tendency toward conflict with other members over how the P.S. Club should operate led him to intermittently abandon these roles. Joe's involvement in leadership roles was also discouraged by other leaders of the club who had grown weary of his involvement. Such conflict is not uncommon in mutual support group contexts (Chien, Norman, & Thompson, 2006; Mohr, 2004). Not everyone wants to get involved in leadership roles, however, including Kevin and Laura, who are not interested despite the P.S. Club welcoming their involvement.

Component Three: Resource Exchange

All informants regularly exchanged social support in their friendship roles at the P.S. Club. They gave each other someone to play games with, someone to share stories with, and someone who can relate to their mental health problems. Being able to maintain gratifying friendships and recreational experiences allowed members to relieve stress and have fun. In addition, the life histories of Nick, Mary, Sue, and Carl describe the development of paid leadership roles, where informants exchanged their time and energy for financial compensation. These leadership roles also helped participants develop a sense of equality in giving and taking. All friendship and leadership roles were voluntary, which minimized power differentials, imbalanced exchanges, exploitation, and the use of force.

Component Four: Self-Appraisal

When all seven of the CRO informants were involved in the CRO, all seven appeared to be benefiting from positive self-appraisal. All seven have memories of good times at the CRO, where everyone was laughing, reflecting positive appraisals back to everyone else. The emotional supports exchanged during these good times led informants to feel good about themselves and accepted at P.S. Club. In this sense, the fun of CRO-related recreation is not just for fun but also for self-esteem. Furthermore, Nick, Sue, Mary, and Carl obtained positive self-appraisals in their leadership roles. Successfully performing tasks related to these helper roles enabled the generation of positive self-appraisals among informants, such as feeling valued and useful.

Component Five: Building Role Skills

Some informants developed new skills. Nick developed accounting and public speaking skills in his role as director. Sue developed problem-solving skills in her leadership roles and Carl developed social skills in the friendship roles he never had as a child. However, Kevin, Laura, Joe, and Mary did not attribute any skill developments to their involvement in the P.S. Club. It may be that the roles these informants maintained at the P.S. Club were familiar enough that new skills did not need to be developed in order to meet role expectations. Although skill development cannot be expected of all CRO participants, it may consistently occur when people take on unfamiliar roles. Nick, Carl, and Sue all developed new skills from new roles.

Component Six: Identity Transformation

The welcoming atmosphere of the P.S. Club helped all informants develop a sense of belonging at the club and embrace the identity of P.S. Club member. Five of the seven informants also developed an increased sense of independence. The social support available at the CRO helped Laura become less dependent on her parents. Mary and Carl felt the social support helped them become less dependent on psychiatric hospitalization when crises arose. Sue reached financial independence because of the full time job she obtained. Her prior CRO leadership involvement helped to prepare her for the job. Nick is also more financially independent because of the money he receives as director of the P.S. Club and more generally independent because he has transitioned out of dependency roles with his parents and his therapist.

Those informants who developed new skills also experienced related identity transformations. Carl developed social skills and began to see himself as a sociable person. Nick and Sue developed skills related to their leadership involvement. Nick and Sue also came to see themselves as leaders and role models for others with mental health problems.

Limitations and Future Research

One shortcoming of this study is its retrospective design. To tell their life histories, participants recalled information from many years ago. As a result, recall bias is a major concern in judging the quality of the data collected. However, this study is interested in understanding how CRO participation is beneficial *from the perspective of informants*, thus reducing the significance of recall bias. The reconstructive bias is an integral aspect of understanding the current perspectives of CRO participants.

Another weakness of this study is that the data do not capture the many people who join a CRO and quit soon thereafter. Recruiting and keeping people involved is a major challenge for CROs. Why some people quit after attending a CRO a few times although others increase their involvement is an important research question that needs to be addressed in other CRO studies.

Although the role framework was able to capture a variety of changes experienced by informants, more research is needed to understand how frequently different benefits are experienced. Future quantitative work can simultaneously test the accuracy of the theoretical framework and evaluate the effectiveness of CROs.

Conclusion

The life histories reflect numerous benefits of CRO participation. The theoretical framework enables organization of those benefits into a coherent framework. Through participation in a welcoming setting, informants developed friendship and leadership roles. In these helper roles, participants exchanged social support and contributed to organizational functioning. Success in meeting helper role expectations enabled the attainment of positive appraisals from both self and others. These positive appraisals promoted emotional well-being and self-esteem. However, informants often had to build new skills in order to be successful. The challenges and triumphs of these new roles frequently led to identity transformations such as an increased sense of independence. No longer trapped in dependency roles, participants began "making it sane" as independent citizens valued by others.

Chapter 7
How Organizations Influence Role Development

Abstract This chapter examines the influence of organizational characteristics on role and relationship development within mental health consumer-run organizations (CROs). The ideas of behavior setting theory and the role framework guide the investigation. Specifically, the chapter examines the influence of organizational size on person–environment interaction and the subsequent development of leadership roles. The chapter also examines how the availability of leadership roles within a CRO relates to recovery progress among members. These relations are tested using data from 250 participants at 20 CROs in multilevel regression analyses. Results provide insight into the strengths and weaknesses of behavior setting theory and the role framework. Together, the two theories inform one another to enhance understanding of CROs.

This chapter and the next chapter provide quantitative analyses that explore relations between role framework components. The current chapter examines how characteristics of the environment influence person–environment interaction, subsequent role and relationship development, and recovery. More specifically, first goal of the chapter is to improve understanding of how organizational size influences person–environment interaction and subsequent involvement in leadership roles. Understanding the impact of size on CRO functioning and determining the optimal size of a CRO will inform decisions about how many consumers are needed to form an effective organization and when a CRO would be more successful if it split into two organizations.

The second goal of the chapter is to examine whether leadership involvement is the primary means by which CROs promote recovery. If leadership involvement is the root cause of CRO participation benefits, then CRO leaders and policy makers will want to prioritize the encouragement of leadership involvement above other organizational concerns. However, if it is not the primary determining factor, other organizational priorities may take precedence. Following are discussions of organizational size and leadership involvement. The introductory section of this chapter concludes with an explanation of study hypotheses.

Organizational Size

Organizational size is an important environmental characteristic that is known to influence functioning (e.g., Camisón-Zornoza, Lapiedra-Alcamí, Segarra-Ciprés, & Boronat-Navarro, 2004). Within the business organization literature, researchers have examined the relationship between size and several facets of organizational functioning (e.g., Blau, 1970; Dewar & Hage, 1978). Although this research base has merit, it has limited applicability to CROs and other small nonprofits because a small for-profit company is equal in size to a large nonprofit organization that relies heavily on volunteer support.

Work from the voluntary nonprofit sector is more relevant to CROs. Smith (2000) theorizes that as organizational size increases, centralization of decision making will also increase. Reaching consensus becomes more difficult as the number of members involved in decision making increases. Thus, organizations typically limit the number of individuals involved in organizational decision making in order to expedite decision-making processes and remain capable of adjusting to changing external circumstances.

The underpopulation and overpopulation hypotheses from behavior setting theory make the same prediction, but provide a richer conceptual understanding of how increases in the number of members influence person–environment interaction (Schoggen, 1989). The application of these hypotheses to CROs presents a quandary in identifying the optimal size of CROs. Both small and large organizations have advantages that are important for organizational success.

The overpopulation hypothesis states that in an optimally populated or overpopulated setting, there are more members available than there are roles to fill. Because there are plenty of members, settings select only the most capable to fill organizational roles, excluding other less capable members. When behavior settings become too overpopulated "vetoing circuits" are frequently used to exclude people from the behavior setting.

Previous research suggests that a strong leadership base is critical to operating an effective CRO (Kaufmann et al., 1993). In developing a strong leadership base, an overpopulated behavior setting is advantageous because it allows vetoing circuits to operate, excluding the weaker candidates from leadership positions. As a result overpopulated CROs will have a surplus of capable leaders operating a productive organization.

Leadership Involvement

An overpopulated setting appears to be the ideal scenario until one considers those members who are being excluded from leadership roles. Although involving everyone in organizational planning and decision making is held as an ideal within CROs that value a participatory process, having everyone involved in all organizational decisions becomes cumbersome. As a result, CROs are likely to maintain a limited number of leadership roles in which people are significantly contributing to organizational planning and decision making.

As discussed in previous chapters and described by the role framework, involvement in leadership roles is a critical avenue by which people benefit from CRO participation. The development of leadership roles enables resource exchanges, where leaders expend time and energy resources on activities that enhance CRO success. In return, leaders receive positive appraisals from fellow members who appreciate their efforts. In a paid leadership position, leaders also receive financial compensation for their efforts. Many of the rewards of leadership involvement are intrinsic, however. Members who value contribution to society can enhance their self-appraisals through volunteer contribution. CRO leaders can also develop news skills when their leadership involvement pushes them to take on unfamiliar tasks. Finally, CRO members who take on leadership roles for an extended period of time may experience identity transformation and begin to view themselves as leaders, seeking similar leadership roles in other community settings. Consistent with the idea that leadership involvement is critical to a beneficial CRO participation experience, previous research found that involvement in CRO operations was the best predictor of personal empowerment and social functioning (Segal & Silverman, 2002).

If there are a limited number of CRO leadership roles, but it is these leadership roles that promote recovery, then underpopulated settings appear to be ideal for facilitating recovery. Underpopulated settings have more roles than members, making every member essential (Barker, 1968; Schoggen, 1989). In underpopulated settings, environmental opportunities to develop new skills are plentiful. Rather than exclude people through "vetoing circuits," underpopulated settings use "deviation-countering circuits" to help people learn the correct behavior.

Recovery

Although leadership involvement could influence a variety of CRO participation outcomes, this study focuses on the concept of recovery as a participation outcome. Chapter 2 provides a traditional definition of recovery, describing it as an ongoing process that emphasizes the self-determined cultivation of the knowledge, skills, and coping abilities needed to live a meaningful, satisfying life (Anthony, 1993). Rather than reach a biological state absent of disease, people learn to manage their mental health problems, taking advantage of useful helping resources in a self-directed manner, so that they can live a hopeful life that does not revolve around their mental health problems (Deegan, 1988; Noordsy et al., 2002).

The current chapter provides a more focused and concrete conceptualization of recovery, defining it as a problem-solving process, where people build capacity in order to overcome stressors and achieve wellness-enhancing goals. In other words, recovery is improved problem solving or coping ability that promotes well-being.

People can recover previous states of wellness by overcoming stressors through problem solving. Similarly, people can create new states of wellness by developing new capacities that can be used to achieve new goals.

Some notions of recovery in the literature are similar to this conceptualization. For example, Deegan (1988, p. 15) describes recovery as the "real life experience of persons as they accept and overcome the challenge of the disability." Other notions of recovery use different words to describe the same basic notion. For example, Noordsy et al. (2002) propose three criteria to define recovery: hope, self-responsibility, and "getting on with life" beyond illness. The notion of recovery as improved coping embodies these concepts. Active problem solving cannot occur if a person does not take responsibility for the consequences of his or her own actions. Setting goals is another essential element of the problem-solving process that provides people with hope. When people begin to problem solve in areas of life separate from their symptoms, they begin to "get on with life" beyond illness. Conceptualizing recovery as a problem-solving process, where individual capacity is employed to achieve wellness enhancing goals, provides a robust but precise understanding of the term recovery.

Study Hypotheses

This study tests two hypotheses related to the predictions of behavior setting theory. The first hypothesis states that as the organizational size of a CRO increases, the proportion of members involved in organizational planning and decision making within the organization decreases. That is, in overpopulated settings, more members will be excluded from CRO leadership roles. Although increasing organizational size is hypothesized to create a more competitive setting, behavior setting theory still acknowledges that the number of roles available does increase as the size of the behavior setting increases. Thus, the second hypothesis states that organizational size will be positively related to the number of members contributing to organizational planning and management.

The relation between organizational size and leadership involvement is particularly important if leadership involvement is the primary means by which people benefit from CROs. The third hypothesis states that as the proportion of members involved in leadership roles increases, the average level of recovery attributed to CRO participation will increase. This hypothesis is based on the work of Segal and Silverman (2002), who found that getting involved in the organizational operations and decision making was the strongest predictor of CRO participation benefits.

Method

To test the above hypotheses, this study analyzes the organizational characteristics of the 20 CROs described in Chap. 3. Organizational data was collected from three sources: quarterly reports submitted to the funding agency, an organizational activity survey completed by organizational leaders, and an organizational health survey completed by CRO leaders and regular members. Following is further information about each of the three data sources and the measures used in this study.

CRO Quarterly Reports

Like other nonprofits who receive public funding, CROs are required to submit quarterly reports. This study analyzes each CRO's second quarter report from fiscal year 2004 (10/1/2003–12/31/2003). Data subject to analysis in these quarterly reports was the unduplicated count of members who attended the CRO during the quarter. This number represents the variable organizational size.

Organizational Activity Survey

Information about leadership roles was collected through an organizational activity survey (see Appendix B) administered to one or more CRO leaders, such as the executive director, who would work together to complete one survey for each CRO. Surveys were completed either in person during the site visits or through telephone interviews. Data for this study came from two survey questions.

The first question asked respondents to report the approximate number of CRO members involved in reporting and management (this includes completing quarterly reports, grants, tax reporting, budget management, and hiring decisions). The second question asked respondents to approximate the number of members involved in planning and organizing all of the different CRO activities. Although approximations were provided, estimates were relatively specific, such as 4–6 or 7–9 people. These two questions are used to measure the number of people involved in organizational planning and decision making, which served as an approximation of the number of leadership roles in an organization: the members in these roles have a major influence on organizational operations, frequently working as members of the board of directors or paid staff. The members in these leadership roles dominate the participatory decision-making process.

Organizational Health Survey

Chapter 3 provides a description of the study sample and data collection procedure for the organizational health survey (Appendix A). Although the organizational health survey collected data on many facets of CRO participation, the current study only used data from a measure of recovery. The 15-item scale asked for participant's perceptions of how they have changed since becoming involved in the CRO.

Table 7.1 Progress towards recovery attributable to CRO participation ($N=250$)

Since I have become involved here…	% Who agree or strongly agree
I feel better about myself	81
I have become more confident	81
I am better able to control my life	77
I have become more competent	75
I have become more independent	74
I have become more effective in getting what I need	74
I deal more effectively with daily problems	74
I do better in social situations	73
I am better able to deal with a crisis	71
I have become more ambitious	70
I do better with my leisure time (i.e., I get more out of leisure time)	70
I can deal better with people and situations that used to be a problem for me	68
I am getting along better with my family	65
My symptoms are not bothering me as much	61
I do better in school or work. (if applicable)	55

Individual items focus on coping abilities such as dealing with a crisis, getting along with family, and managing symptoms. Additionally, items reflecting self-image as it relates to coping were included, such as perceived competence, confidence, and self-esteem. The scale was based on the "Consumer Satisfaction Survey" developed by the Mental Health Statistics Improvement Program (MHSIP, 2000; Teague, Ganju, Hornik, Johnson & McKinney 1997). The modified scale used seven items from the MSHIP, along with five items added to the scale in the common protocol of the Consumer Operated Services Program (COSP 2000) and three items constructed by researchers at the Center for Community Support and Research (Brown et al., 2007b). The scale demonstrated high reliability ($\alpha=0.94$), which is similar to the alphas of 0.91 and 0.98 reported by Teague et al. (1997). Respondents answered questions on a five-point scale ranging from *strongly disagree* to *strongly agree*. A list of all questions in this scale is presented in Table 7.1. To compute an overall scale score, the results from individual items were summed for each respondent. To represent the average member's recovery progress for each CRO, I computed the mean of all scale scores from that CRO. All analyses took place at the organizational level, with an N of 20.

Results

Survey results on recovery attributable to CRO participation are generally positive. Over half of respondents either agreed or strongly agreed with all 15 statements. Table 7.1 provides a summary of the results from this scale. Table 7.2 provides descriptive statistics for all measures used in correlation analysis, along with the

Results

Table 7.2 Mean, standard deviation, and range of all variables under study ($N=20$)

Variable name	Mean	Standard deviation	Range
Organizational size	58.4	50.7	9–171
Organizational planning/management size	15.5	8.5	4–35
Percent members in planning/management	38%	21%	09–85
Recovery	3.8	0.24	3.3–4.2

Table 7.3 Correlations between primary variables under study ($N=20$)

Variable name	(1)	(2)	(3)
(1) Organizational size	–		
(2) Organizational planning and management size	0.74**	–	
(3) Percent members in planning/management	−0.65**	−0.12	–
(4) Recovery	0.38	0.55*	−0.16

*$p<0.05$, **$p<0.01$

mean and standard deviation of each measure. Table 7.3 provides a correlation matrix of the four primary measures used in analysis (1) organizational size (total number of CRO members); (2) organizational planning and management size (number of members involved in planning and management); (3) percent members in planning/management; and (4) recovery attributable to CRO participation.

In its simplest form, correlation analysis indicates congruence with the underpopulation and overpopulation behavior setting hypotheses. Just as the underpopulation/overpopulation hypothesis would predict, smaller organizations have a larger percentage of members involved in planning/management than larger organizations. As the organizational size of a CRO increases, the percentage of members contributing to organizational management decreases ($r=-0.60$, $p<0.01$, $r^2=0.36$). In line with this finding is the negative correlation between organizational size and the percentage of members contributing to the planning and organization of activities ($r=-0.50$, $p<0.05$, $r^2=0.25$). Although duplication of members cannot be accounted for, when these two measures are summed and correlated with organizational size, the negative relationship becomes even stronger ($r=-0.65$, $p<0.01$, $r^2=0.42$). These separate correlations all indicate that as organizational size increases, the percentage of members excluded from leadership roles increases.

Although increasing organizational size provides diminishing returns in the percentage of members contributing to organizational planning/management, the number of members contributing to organizational management still increases as organizational size increases ($r=0.46$, $p<0.05$, $r^2=0.21$). In line with this finding is the correlation between organizational size and the number of members contributing to the planning and organizing of activities ($r=0.73$, $p<0.001$, $r^2=0.53$). Again, when these two leadership size measures are summed, they retain a strong correlation with organizational size ($r=0.74$, $p<0.001$, $r^2=0.55$). Behavior setting

Table 7.4 Regression predicting recovery ($N=250$ individuals, 20 CRO clusters)

Predictor name	Estimate	Standard error
Organizational size	−0.26	0.15
Organizational planning and management size	0.38**	0.10
Percent members in planning/management	−0.19	0.12

**$p<0.01$

Table 7.5 Regression predicting recovery ($N=250$ individuals, 20 CRO clusters)

Predictor name	Estimate	Standard error
Organizational planning and management size	0.21**	0.06
Percent members in planning/management	−0.05	0.07

**$p<0.01$

theory predicts these correlations, stating that the number of roles in a behavior setting increases along with the number of people available to operate the setting, only at a slower rate.

Although findings are congruent with the expectations of behavior setting theory, they are incongruent with the predictions of Segal and Silverman (2002). The hypothesis that recovery will decrease as involvement in organizational planning and decision making decreases was not supported. Instead, results indicate a nonsignificant correlation in the direction opposite of the hypothesis ($r=-0.16$, $p=0.49$).

To further explore the relation between the percentage of members in planning/management and recovery, I estimated regression models in SAS 9.2. Initially, I estimated multilevel random intercept models using Proc Mixed to account for the nesting of individuals within CROs. However, the random intercept variance was not significant, so I switched to Proc Surveyreg, which adjusts standard errors to account for the nested data without estimating a random intercept. Table 7.4 presents results from the initial regression model, which used organizational size, organizational planning and management size, and percent members in planning/management as predictors of recovery. All variables are standardized. Results do not support the third hypothesis. A one-standard deviation (SD) increase in the percentage of members involved in planning/management predicts a nonsignificant −0.19 SD decrease in recovery. However, a one SD increase in organizational planning and management size (an increase of 8.5 members) predicts an increase of 0.38 SD in recovery progress.

Results suggest the multicollinearity between organizational size and organizational planning and management size may be causing unstable estimates; organizational size predicted a decrease in recovery attributable to CRO participation in the model despite having a positive zero-order correlation with recovery. Thus, Table 7.5 presents regression results after removing organizational size as a predictor. Findings remained substantively the same, but with a smaller magnitude. A one SD increase in organizational planning and management size predicts a 0.21 SD increase in recovery.

Discussion

Whereas the results provide insight into the validity of the three hypotheses, the discussion explores how results speak to the two goals of the chapter. Explored first is the question of how organizational size influences leadership role development. Second is a discussion of how leadership role development relates to recovery. Finally, the chapter concludes with a discussion of how combined consideration of behavior setting theory and the role framework can improve the explanatory power of both perspectives.

How Organizational Size Influences Leadership Role Development

Results suggest that as CROs become larger, there is a decline in the percentage of members contributing to organizational planning and management. According to behavior setting theory, this is because it becomes increasingly competitive to get involved in these leadership roles. Larger CROs appear to be facing overpopulated conditions, where vetoing circuits are effectively used to exclude some members from leadership positions. Similar to the selection of varsity athletes in large schools, large CROs have the luxury of being able to select only the most qualified members for paid positions. Large CROs additionally benefit from the most motivated volunteers naturally working their way into leadership positions. One example is the surplus of candidates that sometimes compete to be elected to board officer positions in large organizations, while small organizations often struggle to simply find enough people willing to take on the board officer positions.

Overpopulated CROs are not only able to select the most competent leaders, but they also benefit from having more leaders overall. Although the size of the organization has a strong influence on the percentage of members involved in operating the organization, there remains a strong positive relationship between organizational size and the number of people involved in organizational planning and management ($r=0.74$, $p<0.001$). This correlation is important because previous research found CRO leadership size was positively associated with organizational productivity (Brown 2004). Additionally, research by Kaufmann et al. (1993) found that a large leadership base is critical to successful organizational functioning. Based on these studies, it appears that large CROs are more likely to be successful in the long term because they have more leaders.

Members of smaller CROs may also be more likely to face burnout from taking on too many organizational roles. If a leader from an underpopulated CRO leaves, the existence of the CRO is more likely to be threatened. The engagement of new leaders becomes critical to the survival of the organization. For example, the P.S. Club has been very stable over the years despite its small size. However, if Nick suddenly left the organization, its survival would be threatened because his efforts are central to the P.S. Club's success.

How Leadership Role Development Influences Recovery

Although larger organizations have a smaller percentage of members involved in leadership roles, the smaller percentage does not appear to negatively impact the organization's ability to facilitate recovery. As the percentage of members in planning and management roles decreases, the average level of progress towards recovery increases ($r=-0.16$, $p=0.49$). Although the correlation and subsequent regression estimates were not significant, they were in the opposite direction of the hypothesis, which was based on the empirical work of Segal and Silverman (2002). Clearly, there is some other, more powerful mechanism causing average member's progress towards recovery.

This raises the question of what people who are not in leadership roles are doing while they are participating in CROs. Instead of leading the organization towards productivity, these individuals are enjoying the multitude of activities offered by CROs. They are making friends, forming mutually supportive relationships, and contributing to the organization through support roles.

The improved social networks and social support that are derived from CRO participation may be enabling recovery. Mowbray and Tan (1993) found that social support was the dominant reason for members' continued participation in CROs. The existence of social support has been linked to a variety of mental and physical health outcomes including recovery from chronic diseases, greater life satisfaction, enhanced ability to cope with life stressors, improvement in mental health symptoms, and an overall ability to function in instrumental roles (Cohen et al., 2000; Cohen & Wills, 1985; Thoits, 2010).

Intertwined with social support is the existence of mutually supportive relationships in which people play the roles of both help receiver and help provider. As discussed in the role framework, these mutually supportive exchanges can increase resource acquisition, enhance self-appraisals, promote skill development, and lead to identity transformations. It may be that the socially supportive friendship roles developed through CRO participation are central to recovery because they promote the most beneficial resource exchanges, self-appraisals, skill developments, and identity transformations. Both organizational leaders and the general membership can benefit from mutually supportive friendships formed at the CRO.

Although the development of socially supportive friendship roles may be central to recovery progress within a CRO, results from this study do not provide empirical support for this explanation. Results only suggest that involvement in a leadership role within a CRO is not the *primary* mechanism by which members benefit from participation. Involvement in leadership roles may still be a secondary mechanism facilitating recovery. The positive relationship between organizational decision making and positive individual outcomes found by Segal and Silverman (2002) is likely to be accurate. Their study had no measure of social support or mutually supportive relationships formed; thus organizationally mediated empowerment had no other powerful predictors to compete with. For this reason, the importance of a participatory process within CROs should not be ignored, only moderated.

It is important to note that although the *percentage* of members involved in organizational planning and management does not predict enhanced progress towards recovery, the overall *number* of members involved in organizational planning and management is associated with increased progress towards recovery ($r=0.55$, $p<0.05$). This positive association persisted after controlling for the influence of organizational size and the percentage of members involved in planning/ management in a regression model (see Table 7.4). As such, it appears important for CROs to encourage involvement in leadership roles regardless of whether the involvement itself enhances recovery.

Organizations with more leaders may be able to offer higher quality opportunities for social engagement. By having more paid staff and more voluntary leadership, larger organizations can keep CROs open longer hours while providing a richer diversity of activities that facilitate the development of mutually supportive relationships. Thus, organizations with more leaders may not only be more stable, but also better able to support recovery.

Shortcomings of Behavior Setting Theory

Although the results were congruent with the predictions of behavior setting theory in the sense that leadership roles did become overpopulated, the organizations as a whole did not appear to be overpopulated. Instead, individuals not involved in leadership roles appear to be getting involved in recreational activities and friendship roles. It may be that as leadership roles become overpopulated, the CRO as a whole approaches optimal population. Just as public spaces and other settings that emphasize unstructured socialization reach optimal population when they are crowded (Whyte, 1980), CROs may provide a more attractive social setting when they are crowded on a regular basis.

The underpopulation and overpopulation hypotheses lack explanatory power because they do not consider the idea that some roles within a behavior setting may be overpopulated while others are underpopulated. In any behavior setting, there can be too few or too many individuals trying to occupy a specific role. For example, a newspaper can have too many editors and not enough writers. While these two positions require similar skill sets, the people in each of these roles are not always interested in switching roles. Newsrooms and other behavior settings are frequently underpopulated with respect to a specific role even though the setting as a whole may have a surplus of members. By examining which roles exist within an organization and how many people need to be in each role, a more accurate conceptualization of under and overpopulated behavior settings can be obtained.

Integrating the Role Framework and Behavior Setting Theory

Considered together, the role framework and behavior setting theory inform one another, providing a more comprehensive understanding of CROs and other community settings. As previously discussed, concepts from behavior setting theory enhance understanding of how person–environment interaction leads to role and relationship development. Here, I discuss how consideration of roles can provide insight into the nature of behavior settings.

A key advantage of the concept of roles is that they can be defined as broadly or as specifically as is useful in understanding a setting. To understand a CRO, one may want to focus only on leadership and friendship roles. However, a more fine grained analysis is possible. It may be that different leadership roles have different consequences. For example, being in a paid leadership position may have different consequences that being in a voluntary leadership position. Similarly, the role of president, treasurer, and secretary on the board of directors may lead to the development of different resource exchanges, skills, and self-appraisals. As more roles are taken into consideration, we will obtain a richer description of the standing behavior pattern. Likewise, an understanding of all the different roles played by an individual provides insight into who that person is and what skills they possess.

The addition of roles as a unit of measurement in behavior settings accomplishes several goals that other similar extensions have addressed. Wicker, McGrath, & Armstrong (1972) suggested refining the underpopulation and overpopulation hypotheses to take into consideration the difference in population levels between people who have positions of responsibility and those who are merely members, clients, or onlookers. For example, a restaurant can have too many patrons and not enough staff or vice versa. While Wicker et al. did not explicitly use the concept of roles, their refinement represents a specialized extension of the more generalized expansion suggested here.

Wicker (1991) also suggests the use of cognitive scripts to understand behavior settings. Scripts are cognitive structures that describe appropriate sequences of events in a particular context (Schank & Abelson, 1995). A script can be thought of as the sum of role expectations an individual has both for themselves and all other actors in a behavior setting. While cognitive scripts provide an accurate description of how people conceptualize setting programs, they are not useful as a unit of analysis the way roles are.

How the Role Framework Can Address Several Criticisms of Behavior Setting Theory

One major criticism of behavior setting theory is that it does not meaningfully integrate any individual difference factors (Perkins, Burns, Perry, & Nielsen, 1988).

The integration of the role framework can help to address this issue. Because people selectively interact with behavior settings to fill roles that match their identity, certain people are likely to be drawn to certain settings where they can fulfill certain roles.

Behavior setting theory is also criticized for being a unidirectional model, where settings influence people but people do not influence settings (Perkins et al., 1988). The role framework facilitates understanding of the interaction between settings and people. People are likely to structure settings around roles they are familiar with. Once these roles are entrenched, settings will be most welcoming to people who fill those roles. For example, people who prefer authoritarian roles are likely to set up organizations that have a rigid hierarchy. Once this authoritarian structure is established, the addition of individuals who prefer a more egalitarian, collaborative approach will cause tension, and the newcomers will probably either change the setting or leave the setting.

Criticism has also risen over behavior setting theory's inability to account for the personal satisfaction derived from participation in a behavior setting (Perkins et al., 1988). If practitioners want to make behavior settings more rewarding and beneficial to participants, then they will need to understand how involvement in the setting can be personally satisfying. The role framework provides a strong theoretical link between the properties of behavior settings and how people may benefit from participation in these settings. The roles available in a setting provide insight into what resource exchanges, skills, and identities people are likely to develop in that setting.

Limitations and Future Research

One of the major limitations of the study presented in this chapter is its reliance on correlations between variables in drawing conclusions. Although correlations indicate a relationship between variables, they do not indicate a causal relationship. We cannot rule out the possibility that an entirely different set of causal relationships is operating. Additionally, results are based on a small sample size and some relationships found in the data may be unique to CROs in Kansas; this limits the generalizability of findings. Finding significance with a small sample size requires relatively strong relations between variables, however, and these relationships are likely to remain significant with larger sample sizes, even if the magnitude of the relations are not as large as was found in this study.

One area clearly in need of additional quantitative research is how different roles available in a CRO relate to recovery. Although leadership involvement is unlikely to be the primary mechanism by which CROs promote recovery, it may still contribute to recovery.

Conclusions

With respect to the question of how organizational size influences role development in a CRO, it appears that there is an upper limit to the number of members who can get involved in leadership roles. However, larger CROs still have a larger number of leaders, which appears to be important not only for organizational productivity but also organizational ability to promote recovery. Additionally, larger CROs can still engage members in various organizational activities and fill support roles, such as help with building maintenance. With respect to the question of how CRO participants make recovery progress, it does not appear that engagement in a leadership role is the primary force contributing to recovery. Instead, it may be the benefits derived from the formation of socially supportive friendship roles.

Results also reveal weaknesses in the underpopulation and overpopulation hypotheses' ability to account for the intricacies of behavior settings. Larger CROs appear to be overpopulated with respect to leadership roles but adequately populated with respect to other organizational roles. Consideration of the role framework helps to account for this finding and extend the explanatory power of behavior setting theory. Usage of the role concept helps to provide a rich description of a setting's standing behavior pattern, while also providing insight into how different roles lead to different benefits. Researchers, practitioners, and policy makers can use this extension to create and modify behavior settings so its inhabitants will develop new patterns of resource exchange, alter their self-appraisals, learn new skills, and develop identities that promote health.

Chapter 8
Role Development and Recovery

Abstract When people participate in mental health consumer-run organizations (CROs), they frequently develop socially supportive friendship roles, empowering leadership roles, or both. The role framework suggests both of these roles can lead to a variety of participation benefits. This chapter presents results from a study examining the differential influence of these two types of roles on recovery. In an analysis of 250 CRO members from 20 CROs, the study uses structural equation modeling to examine the relationship between role involvement and recovery. Findings indicate both roles are related to recovery, however socially supportive friendship roles have a stronger relationship than empowering leadership roles. Discussion focuses on how CROs can promote the development of a socially supportive and empowering environment.

In the previous chapter, I discussed two types of involvement in CROs: leadership roles and friendship roles. Although more fine-grained distinctions are possible, these two roles provide a parsimonious description of CRO involvement. From a theoretical perspective, each role provides unique benefits. Empowerment theory explains how leadership roles can promote recovery, whereas the social support literature explains how friendship roles can impact recovery (Helgeson & Gottlieb, 2000; Holter et al., 2004; Maton & Salem, 1995; Nelson et al., 2001; Segal et al., 1993). The relative impact these two types of roles have in promoting recovery is not understood. The goal of the current chapter is to understand the extent to which involvement in socially supportive friendship roles and empowering leadership roles contributes to recovery in the CRO context.

Understanding how socially supportive friendship roles and empowering leadership roles influence recovery is important because numerous CRO members experience either socially supportive friendship roles or empowering leadership roles but not both. If only one of these types of participation is related to recovery, then progress toward recovery can only be expected from a subgroup of all CRO participants. Furthermore, this knowledge can be used to guide CRO practice. Understanding which types of CRO role development influence recovery informs organizational leaders about the types of involvement their CRO should encourage.

Role Development and Recovery

Previous chapters have described how the development of socially supportive friendship roles and empowering leadership roles can enable (1) beneficial resource exchanges; (2) enhanced self-appraisals; (3) skill development; and (4) identity transformation. Each of these four consequences of role and relationship development described by the role framework are theorized to impact progress toward recovery, as discussed further in Chaps. 2 and 3.

The current study focuses explicitly on the link between role development and recovery. More specifically, the current study focuses on understanding the difference between developing socially supportive friendship roles and empowering leadership roles in making recovery progress that is attributable to CRO participation. A socially supportive friendship role generally involves the development of friendships through participation in social activities at the CRO, whereas an empowering leadership role involves contributions to organizational operations and decision making. Recovery is conceptualized as the development of problem solving and coping skills to achieve wellness enhancing goals, as further described in Chap. 7.

Chapter 2 provides a description of how social support and empowerment processes are theorized to promote recovery in the CRO context. Specifically, social support helps buffer stress by providing people with coping resources and enables the direct production of positive affect (Cohen et al., 2000). Although it is clear that socially supportive friendship roles can promote well-being, it is also clear that social relationships do not always promote well-being. For example, relationships high in conflict or coercion can be detrimental to well-being (Rook, 1990, 1992). The conditions under which social relationships contribute to well-being are not easily identified (Thoits, 1985). This study focuses on the attainment of social support in a specific condition – that of CRO participation. It investigates how the perceived availability of social support within a CRO relates to perceived recovery that is attributable to CRO participation.

It is important to note the unique nature of the relationships available in a CRO. As described in Chap. 2, experiential knowledge about mental health problems acts as a key bonding point in the development of supportive relationships. Sharing similar experiences enables validation, a greater capacity for empathy, and reduced emotional isolation (Borkman, 1999; Cowan & Cowan, 1986; Lieberman, 1993; Rosenberg, 1984; Toseland & Rossiter, 1989). Peers may also be able to share coping and problem solving strategies that they have found useful. Hence, the provision of social support in a CRO may be uniquely effective because of the shared experiential knowledge around mental health problems.

Descriptions of empowering settings in the literature frequently include the maintenance of a socially supportive environment (Segal et al., 1993; Maton & Salem, 1995). Although this inclusion is certainly reasonable, it is not universally acknowledged (e.g., Salzer, 1997) and a consensus definition of empowerment remains elusive (Clark & Krupa, 2002). More central to the empowerment construct is the idea of a participatory process where everyone is involved in decision making (Peterson & Zimmerman, 2004). The works of Segal et al. (1993) and Maton and Salem (1995) remain consistent with this focus, despite their broader conceptualization of empowerment.

For the purposes of conceptual clarity, the study described in this chapter defines an empowering leadership role as only the participatory process where individuals influence decision making and organizational operations. By wielding some influence over the functioning of an organization, members can gain a sense of control and ownership with the organization. This organizationally mediated empowerment can transfer into a sense of personal empowerment (Schulz et al., 1995; Zimmerman & Rappaport, 1988).

Relating Friendship and Leadership Roles

Although socially supportive friendship roles and empowering leadership roles are distinct, the benefits that can be accrued from either can be conceptualized as part of a general change process described by the role framework. Both friendship and leadership roles are helper roles rather than dependency roles. In helper roles, people can develop equitable resource exchanges, receive positive appraisals for their helpful actions, develop new skills to succeed in their helping activities, and begin to see themselves as valuable and capable individuals. In a socially supportive friendship role, people can help others by providing emotional support or ideas about how to solve personal problems. In a leadership role, people can help others by accomplishing organizational tasks that are beneficial to everyone. In either case, the rewards of helping others can be derived. Research indicates the act of helping others can improve self-concept, increase energy levels, and improve physical health (Luks, 1991). Although socially supportive friendship roles and empowering leadership roles can be viewed similarly, they nevertheless provide CRO members with distinct helping opportunities that may differentially contribute to recovery.

Study Overview and Hypotheses

This study directly compares the relative influence of socially supportive friendship roles and empowering leadership roles on recovery. The study hypotheses are (1) both socially supportive friendship roles and empowering leadership roles will be positively associated with recovery; and (2) socially supportive friendship roles will have a stronger relationship with recovery than empowering leadership involvement. The first hypothesis is based on the previously presented research on social support and empowerment, the second hypothesis is based on the previous chapter, which suggested leadership involvement is not the primary process by which members benefit from participation.

Method

To test the above hypotheses, this study analyzes the participation experiences of 250 CRO members from 20 CROs in Kansas. All data come from the Organizational Health Questionnaire (Appendix A). The study setting, study sample, and data collection procedure are all described in the Method section of Chap. 3. The following sections describe the measures and the statistical methods used in this study.

Measures

After answering several demographic questions, survey respondents completed items on several facets of CRO participation. Two questions that provided descriptively informative data about respondent's social networks asked (1) At this place, how many people can you talk to about personal things; and (2) Outside of this place, how many people can you talk to about personal things? Data most relevant to testing the hypotheses came from three scales that measured empowering leadership roles, socially supportive friendship roles, and recovery attributable to CRO participation. The measure of recovery is the same as is described in Chap. 8.

To fully measure role involvement, one must capture both the extent to which an individual engages in behaviors expected of someone in a particular role, as well as the extent to which the environment provides the actor with the expected response. In other words, a role is an exchange, which includes both giving and receiving. Unfortunately, strong quantitative measures of socially supportive friendship roles and empowering leadership roles do not yet exist. As such, this study uses pre-existing measures that approximate role involvement.

The degree to which members developed empowering leadership roles was measured by asking members about the different types of involvement they had in organizational functioning and decision making. Although the measure captures what people are expected to give in an empowering leadership role, it does not capture what people are expected to receive, which would include a degree of influence over the direction of the organization and reflected appraisals that one's contributions are valued by members of the organization.

A modified version of the organizationally mediated empowerment scale was used to capture empowering leadership roles (Segal, Silverman, & Temkin, 1995). The 21-item scale demonstrated excellent reliability, with an observed Cronbach's

Method

alpha of 0.91. This is consistent with previous research, where reported alpha coefficients were 0.87 at baseline and 0.90 at 6 months (Segal et al., 1995). The modified scale used 13 of the same items but removed four that were irrelevant to CRO participation in this sample and added eight items that were more pertinent to the sampled CRO members. Respondents answered "yes" or "no" questions about their involvement in organizational operations.

The degree to which members developed socially supportive friendship roles was measured by asking CRO members about their perception of the degree to which social support is available at their CRO. This measure captures what members receive when they develop socially supportive friendship roles in a CRO, but it does not capture what members give. A more complete measure of socially supportive friendship roles would need to capture the extent to which the member provided other CRO members with support.

The 11-item, 4-alternative, Likert scale used to measure socially supportive friendship roles draws its questions from Mowbray and Tan's (1993) Group Support and Mutual Learning Scale (8 items, $\alpha=0.81$) and the Intimacy and Sharing Scale (5 items, $\alpha=0.70$). Mowbray and Tan (1993) based their items on the Group Environment Scale and the Community Oriented Programs Environment Scale (Moos, 1974; Moos & Humphrey, 1974). The scale used in this study demonstrated strong reliability ($\alpha=0.93$).

Statistical Methods

Structural equation modeling (Ullman, 2001) with item parcels (Kishton & Widaman, 1994) was used to examine the impact of empowering leadership roles and socially supportive friendship roles on recovery. Item parcels are created by dividing the items on a test scale into a small number of mutually exclusive and exhaustive subgroups (Kishton & Widaman, 1994). Each participant then has a score on each subgroup (instead of having one overall score), which allows for the use of latent variables in the model. The latent variables account for measurement error more precisely, which yields more accurate results as compared to models that use overall scale scores (Coffman & MacCallum, 2005). For this specific project, three parcels were created for each scale. Because all items on each scale measured the same construct, scale items were randomly divided among the three parcels of the scale.

A path diagram of the model with item parcels is presented in Fig. 8.1. In the main part of the model, the "socially supportive friendship role" and "empowering leadership role" latent variables lead to the "recovery" latent variable. "Years attended" and "attendance frequency" were also added to the model as potential predictors of recovery. To account for the fact that participants were nested within CROs, parameter standard errors and the goodness-of-fit statistic were adjusted using aggregate analysis (Muthén & Satorra, 1995). This adjustment did not substantively change the results. The model was estimated using Mplus version 5.1

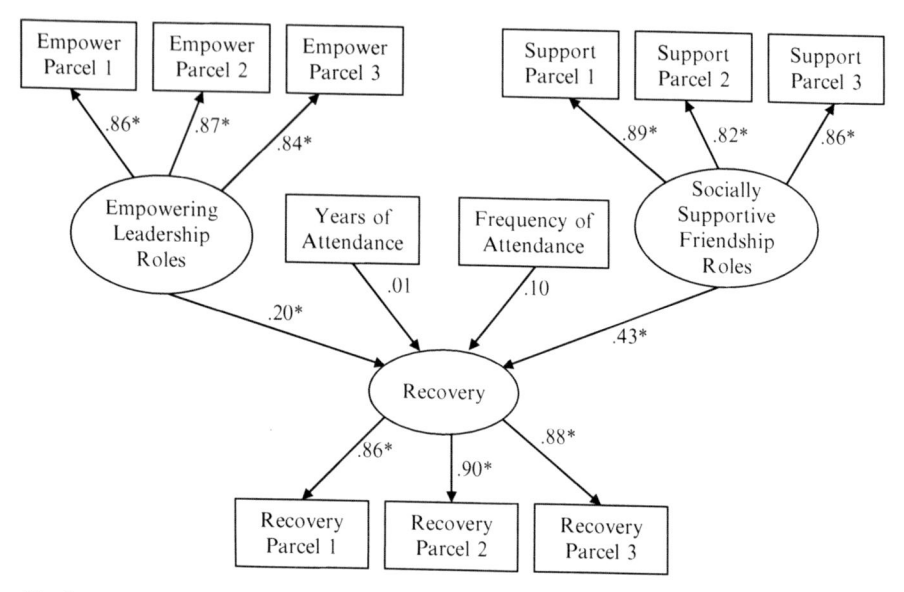

Fig. 8.1 Hypothesized structural equation model with standardized coefficients. For simplicity, neither covariance paths nor errors terms are presented. *$p < 0.01$

(Muthén & Muthén 2007) via the method of full information maximum likelihood (e.g., Wothke, 2000), which has the advantage of being able to handle incomplete data. The proportion of missing data was low (1%), and full information maximum likelihood estimation allowed for the inclusion of these incomplete observations in the model-fitting procedure.

Results

To provide an overview of the results, Fig. 8.1 illustrates the hypothesized structural equation model with control variables and includes standardized regression coefficients. Table 8.1 provides descriptive statistics of the variables used in the model, including the mean, standard deviation, and correlations between variables. The remaining results are divided into three subsections. The first subsection presents results pertinent to the first hypothesis – that both socially supportive friendship roles and empowering leadership roles will be associated with recovery. The second subsection explores the second hypothesis – that socially supportive friendship roles have a stronger relationship with recovery than empowering leadership roles. Finally, in an effort to understand why socially supportive friendship roles are related to recovery, the third subsection describes the social networks of CRO members and how CRO participation changed those networks.

Results

Table 8.1 Means, standard deviations, and correlations between variables in the structural equation model ($N=250$)

Variables	Mean	SD	(1)	(2)	(3)	(4)	(5)	(6)	(7)	(8)	(9)	(10)
(1) Support Parcel 1	9.79	1.89	–									
(2) Support Parcel 2	11.99	2.93	0.73	–								
(3) Support Parcel 3	13.11	2.70	0.77	0.70	–							
(4) Empowerment Parcel 1	3.56	2.08	0.08	0.05	0.06	–						
(5) Empowerment Parcel 2	3.55	2.41	0.02	0.01	0.01	0.75	–					
(6) Empowerment Parcel 3	2.79	1.95	0.06	0.02	0.04	0.73	0.73	–				
(7) Recovery Parcel 1	19.72	3.73	0.36	0.36	0.42	0.19	0.17	0.23	–			
(8) Recovery Parcel 2	18.85	4.02	0.32	0.31	0.32	0.17	0.18	0.22	0.77	–		
(9) Recovery Parcel 3	19.69	4.07	0.35	0.36	0.36	0.21	0.17	0.21	0.75	0.80	–	
(10) Attendance frequency	2.09	0.87	0.07	0.01	-0.03	0.24	0.23	0.24	0.14	0.19	0.09	–
(11) Time attended (years)	0.71	0.34	0.19	0.12	0.10	0.25	0.24	0.15	0.17	0.10	0.13	0.17

Hypothesis 1

Results of the structural equation model support the first hypothesis. There is a positive association between empowering leadership roles and recovery ($z=3.00$, $p<0.05$), suggesting that people who are more involved in the organizational operations of CROs also tend to benefit more from participation. There is also a positive association between socially supportive friendship roles and recovery ($z=5.93, p<0.05$), suggesting that people who experience supportive social involvement also tend to attribute more progress toward recovery as a result of their CRO participation. Finally, the model provides an excellent fit to the data ($\chi^2 (36)=38.7$, $p=0.35$; RMSEA=0.02). This indicates that the relationships specified between variables in the model are plausible, thereby increasing the confidence with which interpretations of the parameter estimates can be made.

It should be noted that we controlled for dosage (years of attendance and frequency of attendance) in the model, in order to ensure that our results indicate the unique outcome variance that cannot be explained by quantity of participation. All of the paths from these covariates to recovery were not significantly different from 0 ($z=0.18$ for years attended; $z=1.01$ for frequency of attendance).

Hypothesis 2

To examine the relative impact of empowering leadership roles and socially supportive friendship roles on recovery, a second model was fit to the data. In this second model, the paths from "empowering leadership roles" and "socially supportive friendship roles" to "recovery" were constrained to be equal. Because this reduced model is nested within the original full model, the fit of the reduced model can be compared to the fit of the full model using the Wald Test of Parameter Constraints (Gourieroux, Holly, & Monfort, 1982). The full model with 36 degrees of freedom fit better than the reduced model with 35 degrees of freedom (Wald test=10.1, $df=1$, $p<0.01$), yielding evidence that the empowering leadership role path is not equal to the socially supportive friendship role path. More specifically, in comparing the standardized regression weights for these paths, it appears that socially supportive friendship roles have a stronger relationship with recovery than do empowering leadership roles. Although both empowering leadership roles and socially supportive friendship roles are positively associated with recovery, the socially supportive friendship roles have a stronger relationship, which is consistent with the second hypothesis.

The Social Networks of CRO Members

Although socially supportive friendship roles appear to be most important in promoting recovery, the reasons why are not fully understood. One possible explanation is that CRO participation allows members to develop larger social networks. Descriptive statistics from the survey provide some insight into the social networks of CRO members and how CRO participation contributes to these social networks.

Comparing the marriage demographics of Kansans using 2000 census data to the marriage demographics of CRO members indicates that CRO members have fewer marriages. Whereas 58% of Kansans over the age of 15 are married only 16% of CRO members are married. Descriptive statistics from the survey also suggest that fellow CRO members are a critical component of the social networks maintained by participants. The average CRO member had 9.7 people who they could talk to about personal matters and 4.7 of those people were fellow CRO members. In other words, 48% of the average CRO member's social network is directly tied to their CRO involvement. It should be noted that 19% of the data on members' social networks were missing. How these missing data affect the results is not known. These questions may have been left blank because it was difficult to estimate the number of people respondents could talk to about personal matters. Questions of this nature are also relatively personal and some people may not have felt comfortable answering them.

Interpretation of Results

Congruent with the first hypothesis, results indicate that both socially supportive friendship roles and empowering leadership roles were related to recovery progress that participants attributed to CRO participation. Appropriate interpretation of the findings requires consideration of how the associational relations identified in this study can be interpreted. The associations found between type of involvement and recovery is congruent with, but not indicative of a causal relationship where involvement leads to recovery. Most likely however, the relationship between involvement and recovery is best described as a two-way interchange. Here the development of socially supportive friendship roles and empowering leadership roles contributes to recovery, while recovery simultaneously promotes role development.

Although firm conclusions cannot be drawn from this observational, cross-sectional study, results are consistent with the idea that encouraging the development of both socially supportive friendship roles and empowering leadership roles will promote the recovery of their members. Creating an environment that encourages socially supportive friendship roles and empowering leadership roles is a challenging task.

The role framework indicates that the development of socially supportive friendship roles and empowering leadership roles depends upon person–environment interaction. CRO environments need to encourage the development of both roles to promote the recovery of their members. In order to promote empowering and supportive organizational environments, the Center for Community Support and Research (CCSR) at Wichita State University has been providing CROs with training and technical assistance for more than a decade. CCSR's work with CROs to improve organizational functioning has led to the identification of several strategies that CROs use to encourage the development of socially supportive friendship roles and empowering leadership roles. Drawing from this experiential knowledge base, the following two sections outline strategies CROs can use to build empowering and socially supportive environments.

Promoting an Empowering Environment

Promoting member involvement in organizational operations is challenging but critical to organizational success, because the task of sustaining a CRO can easily overwhelm a small leadership base. Adding to the challenge is the fact that, in the short term, it often takes longer to train a new individual to complete a task than it does for an experienced individual to complete the task. Once new volunteers gain training and experience however, they can begin to make valuable contributions to the organization independently. Investing in the skill development of volunteers promotes both organizational functioning and an empowering sense of ownership and commitment to the CRO. The learning opportunities may also help members with problem solving in other situations. To avoid replicating a disempowering professional environment where paid staff members take care of consumers, the following subsections discuss several strategies that can help get members contributing to organizational operations early and often.

Volunteer Opportunities

Regularly recruiting members to complete small but recurring organizational duties provides all members with immediate opportunities to contribute to the daily operations of the organization. Through tasks such as meal preparation, transportation assistance, cleaning, and building maintenance, everyone can make substantial contributions to their CRO. The use of sign-up sheets can promote accountability and commitment. Publicly recognizing and rewarding members for their contributions can help to encourage continued volunteerism, enhance camaraderie, and promote the self-esteem of recognized members. Establishing shared social norms with respect to organizational contribution and instilling those attitudes early when members join a CRO can help to get everyone involved.

Organizational Decision Making

Keeping meetings open, encouraging everyone to attend, and seeking the perspectives of all attendees during discussions can improve organizational decision making and help to get all members invested in shaping the policies and practices of their organization. Maintaining nonconfrontational discussions, in which all perspectives are valued can help keep meetings welcoming and productive. Furthermore, when tackling major organizational decisions such as voting for positions on the board of directors, it is especially important to advertise and schedule the meeting at a convenient time. Involving the majority of the members in such decisions is critical to keeping the CRO operating in a manner consistent with the interests and priorities of the general membership.

Planning and Organizing Activities

Providing members with opportunities to plan, organize, and facilitate activities that interest them can be one of the most rewarding voluntary leadership roles offered by CRO. The activities undertaken are only limited by the imagination of members (and the availability of an activity budget) but include game tournaments, group outings, crafts, parties, meals, and learning opportunities (e.g., gardening, cooking, or computer classes). Organizing group activities can be an enjoyable opportunity to develop leadership skills. Forming several small collaborative groups who organize activities on a rotating or ad hoc basis can help to prevent burnout and provide the CRO with a larger pool of members ready to make organizational contributions.

Formal Leadership Positions

CRO participants can also occupy formal leadership roles such as board member, shift manager, or director. These positions typically entail more responsibility and some may require substantial training on topics such as grant writing and completing quarterly reports. Organizations may benefit from spreading a full-time paid staff position across several interested CRO members who can each contribute using their own unique talents. This can help prevent burnout and reliance on a single member. If one paid staff member becomes sick, other experienced staff can temporarily fill in. Another strategy CROs can use to promote shared leadership is to rotate positions on the board of directors every year. This can encourage the development of new leaders and prevent entrenched hierarchies from forming.

Promoting a Socially Supportive Environment

The social support available at a CRO provides a powerful incentive for participation and promotes recovery (Brown, Shepherd, Merkle, Wituk and Meissen 2008; Mowbray & Tan, 1993). In the CRO context, social support may be particularly valuable because members can share experiential knowledge in managing mental health problems. This shared background promotes mutual understanding and empathy

(Borkman, 1999). Organizational leaders can employ several strategies to promote the development of socially supportive friendship roles, as further described in the following sections.

Recognize Member Accomplishments

Recognizing members for their personal accomplishments and contributions can help members develop a sense of self-worth as a capable and valued member of the organization. Furthermore, the act of recognizing member accomplishments can promote mutual affection between the recipient and the recognizer. Accomplishments can be honored through both private interactions (e.g., letters, compliments, tokens of appreciation) and publicly (e.g., banquets, birthday parties). Habitual recognition of member accomplishments by organizational leaders can be particularly effective because CRO leaders have a powerful influence on the atmosphere of the organization. When leaders model supportive interactions, others will often follow their example, enhancing a socially supportive environment.

Organize a Variety of Interesting Activities

By organizing fun and interesting activities, CROs provide a medium for the development of close friendships. Providing members with engaging activities enables comfortable social interaction with reduced pressure to maintain conversation. Although each CRO will want to tailor their activities to the interests of members, some commonly successful activities include holiday parties, crafts, friendly competitions such as pool tournaments, group meals such as potlucks, and field trips. CROs that offer multiple activity options at a given point in time may be the most successful, because members can gravitate toward the activities best suited to their interests while avoiding activities they find boring. Scheduling activities on a weekly basis and mailing a monthly activity calendar to participants can also help regularly attract members who are particularly fond of one activity but otherwise disinclined to participate. Maintaining a dynamic and engaging environment is especially important for attracting and retaining new CRO members because they have not established close relationships with fellow members that can make any activity enjoyable.

Prevent and Resolve Conflict with a Code of Conduct

As with any open social setting, conflicts between members occur at times. If left unchecked, such conflict can negatively impact the well-being of members, deter attendance, erode the socially supportive nature of the CRO, and eventually threaten the existence of the organization (Mohr, 2004). To avoid these consequences, CROs must prioritize conflict prevention and resolution. Developing a code of conduct that provides members with a shared set of behavior expectations during CRO participation can help to prevent and resolve conflicts. For codes of conduct to be effective, all members must be familiar with and accept their content. Effective codes of conduct can develop through group discussions that use consensus-driven decision making to determine acceptable and unacceptable behaviors at the CRO, along with the consequences for violating rules. Revisiting and updating the code of conduct on a regular basis can help maintain member buy-in and ensure new members have the opportunity to influence its content. Within a code of conduct, it can be useful to outline a process for conflict resolution that focuses on addressing the behavior in question rather than criticizing the individual offender. At times, problems may arise that the code of conduct does not address. As such, it may be useful to describe a process for resolving unanticipated problems within the code of conduct.

Develop Self-Help Groups and/or Peer Counselors

Regardless of the self-help group's focal issue, participation encourages mutual self-disclosure and the formation of intimate, trusting relationships between members. The relationship dynamics developed in a self-help group carry over to other CRO activities. The explicit emphasis on sharing personal struggles and mutual encouragement in a self-help group can promote socially supportive exchanges that may not occur in relationships developed through purely social activities. The use of peer counselors is another strategy CROs can use to promote empathic listening and discussions focused on problem solving. The fact that peer counselors have faced similar mental health challenges provides them with a natural strength that nonconsumer counselors do not have. The lived experience of coping with mental health problems can help peer counselors provide practical and appropriate support.

Although the preceding sections have presented numerous strategies for promoting socially supportive and empowering environments, many more yet unmentioned approaches exist. Inevitably, some suggested strategies will work well in some settings and not others; thus, it is important for CROs to consider their own unique situation when selecting strategies. Furthermore, CROs may need to develop entirely new strategies if the proposed strategies prove insufficient. With limited time and resources to devote to any particular challenge or activity, it is important for CROs to find overlap and synergy between efforts to promote empowering leadership roles and socially supportive friendship roles. Balancing both appears to be an important component of effective CRO operation based in the philosophy of recovery.

Comparing Friendship and Leadership Roles

Congruent with the second hypothesis, socially supportive friendship roles maintain a stronger relationship with recovery than empowering leadership roles. This finding is consistent with the previous chapter, which suggested that involvement in organizational planning and decision making was not the primary route by which members made progress toward recovery. Because socially supportive friendship roles maintain a stronger relationship with recovery, it makes sense to prioritize the importance of socially supportive friendship roles when explaining how CRO participation leads to recovery. Developing new socially supportive friendship roles may be a powerful experience for CRO members because of the social isolation they often face prior to CRO involvement.

Marriage demographics are congruent with this notion, as CRO members have substantially fewer marriages than the broader population. Further, results indicate that approximately half of the people CRO members talk to about personal matters are fellow CRO members. The added social support within CROs is likely to have a strong positive influence on member's lives because social support has been linked to a variety of health and mental health outcomes including recovery from chronic diseases, greater life satisfaction, enhanced ability to cope with life stressors, decreased levels of anxiety and depression, and overall ability to function in instrumental roles (Cohen et al., 2000; Cohen & Wills, 1985).

The finding that socially supportive friendship roles have a stronger relationship with recovery than empowering leadership roles has different implications for people interested in the organizational development of CROs. The finding suggests that CROs should prioritize the development of a socially supportive environment over the development of an empowering environment when trying to promote recovery. In other words, limited time and resources may lead CROs to focus on implementing the previously discussed strategies for promoting a socially supportive environment rather than those strategies intended to promote an empowering environment. This is not to say that an empowering environment should always be of secondary concern. At times, it may be easier and thus more efficient to enhance the empowering nature of the CRO environment. Furthermore, if recovery is not the primary concern, then developing a socially supportive environment should not be prioritized over developing an empowering environment. For example, if organizational survival is the primary concern, it may be that an empowering environment should be prioritized because of the organizational contributions that come from empowered members.

Limitations and Future Research

One of the primary limitations of this research is its cross-sectional approach to the study of a longitudinal phenomenon. The process by which members benefit from CRO participation occurs over an extended period of time. While cross-sectional studies can provide some insight into this chronological process, only longitudinal research methods can provide a complete understanding of this change process. Future research may consider a longitudinal cross-lagged structural equation model, where observations at earlier time points are used to predict observations at later time points (Burkholder & Harlow, 2003; Menard, 2002). This type of model could provide insight into the nature of the interaction between individual participation experiences and recovery over time. Additionally, the use of longitudinal multilevel methods, such as a random coefficient model, could provide insight into the relationship between organizational characteristics and individual outcomes (Raudenbush & Bryk, 2002). However, adequate power for statistical inferences at the organizational level may require a sample of at least 100 CROs (Hox & Maas, 2001).

A second limitation of the study is its limited measurement of role involvement. A role is a set of behavioral expectations that describes how people interact with their environment. It is difficult to measure behavioral expectations with precision because people do not always know what is expected of them and what to expect from others, thus requiring improvisation. Improvisation itself is a skill that people refine as they develop a cognitive framework for providing appropriate responses in a particular role. At times, behavioral expectations may be more accurately described as anticipations, predictions, hopes, plans, or assumptions.

With qualitative methods, an individual's own understanding of the role expectations can be assessed. However, quantitative measurement of the degree to which a person has undertaken a particular role requires a priori knowledge of the behavioral expectations associated with the role. In a socially supportive friendship role, behaviors that could be measured include the extent to which an individual shares personal problems, expresses concern, hears potential problem solving strategies, and receives emotional support. Tracking a variety of similar friendship-related behaviors through self-report or behavioral observation could provide a measurement of socially supportive friendships roles that is objectively defined a priori. Unfortunately, such a measure does not yet exist and the current study improvised with a measure of perceived social support that focused on the extent to which the CRO environment was supportive for that individual without considering the socially supportive behaviors of the individual.

The measure of empowering leadership roles focused on counting the number of different leadership activities in which an individual participated. This measure provided an approximation of leadership involvement but it did not capture whether the environmental response was empowering. In other words, it did not capture expectations for the environment in response to the leadership behaviors of the individual. These environmental responses can similarly be measured through behavioral observation or self-report of the frequency with which an actor experiences specific responses. For example, in a leadership role, a person may receive appreciation from group members who benefit from their actions or criticism for performing duties poorly. Thus, what the person receives in their leadership roles determines whether it is empowering. Tracking the patterns of both a person's behavior and the environmental response provides a more complete understanding of the person–environment interactions that make up an empowering leadership role. The measure of socially supportive friendship roles better captures what the environment provides the person, whereas the measure of empowering leadership roles better captures what person provides to the environment.

A third limitation of this study is the predominately Caucasian sample. Whether study findings would generalize to other racial or ethnic groups is not known. Future research using a different sample of CROs is needed to address this question. A fourth limitation of this research has to do not with the study itself but with the discussion of how CROs can promote socially supportive and empowering environments. The proposed strategies for developing these environments are based in extensive experience but not research methods that demonstrate causation. Future research needs to establish best practices for promoting both socially supportive and empowering environments by testing whether the proposed strategies lead to socially supportive or empowering environments.

Finally, experience suggests there may be a common pathway to CRO involvement and leadership. This pathway begins with people becoming socially involved with recreational activities and friendships. Once involved, many people begin volunteering and gradually take on increasing levels of responsibility and leadership. However, the existence of this pathway, how it typically works, and reasons why it often does not, need to be better understood to fully appreciate how socially supportive friendship roles and empowering leadership roles can promote recovery.

Conclusions

When someone joins a CRO, they can get involved in socially supportive friendship roles, empowering leadership roles, or both. This study examined how these two types of roles are related to recovery and found that both maintain a positive association. The relationship between socially supportive friendship roles and recovery is stronger however, which may be due to the social isolation that many people with mental health problems face. CRO participation may help to alleviate this social isolation by increasing participants' social network size. Encouraging social involvement and leadership involvement among CRO members is a critical challenge facing CROs. Numerous strategies exist that CROs can use to develop an environment that encourages both socially supportive friendship roles and empowering leadership roles. The real challenge is implementing these strategies effectively.

Chapter 9
Conclusion

Abstract Drawing from the previously presented life-history narratives of participants in consumer-run organizations (CROs), this chapter seeks to provide general insights into the recovery process. I also consider implications for practice that are based on insights from the role framework and the holistic consideration of all studies presented in the book. The strengths and weaknesses of the qualitative and quantitative methods used to develop and test the role framework are also discussed. Many weaknesses of the qualitative studies are addressed by the quantitative studies and vice versa. However, numerous limitations of the research remain and this chapter presents future research directions that can further improve our understanding of how people benefit from CROs. Finally, the book concludes with some consideration of how the role framework informs future directions for the treatment and prevention of mental health problems.

This concluding chapter seeks to provide readers with insights that cut across several chapters of the book. The first section discusses general insights into the recovery process. The second section summarizes the book's implications for practice and the third discusses the strengths and limitations of the research methods. Following is a section on future research directions that can address identified weaknesses and more rigorously test the predictions of the role framework. Finally, closing remarks consider the future of CROs and the broader implications of the role framework.

General Insights into the Recovery Process

The narratives suggest recovering from severe mental health problems is a lifelong process. Despite remarkable progress, no one reached a point in which their mental health problems stopped being a major life challenge. Thus, the biomedical view of recovery as a return to a biological state absent of disease appears largely unrealistic for people with serious mental health problems. However, the consumer recovery model provides an accurate depiction of the recovery process described in the life-history narratives. Change was gradual, with people losing ground at times. For example, Carl made great progress through his involvement in the Breakthrough House but then suffered a setback because of his failed marriage. As his involvement in the P.S. Club progressed, he not only regained lost ground but continued growing through his leadership involvement. As is typical for people pursuing any life goal, recovery is a nonlinear process where people can take two steps forward and one step back (Chiu, Ho, Lo, & Yiu, 2010).

From the seven narratives, it becomes clear that medications play a critical role in recovery. Clozaril, a second-generation antipsychotic medication, appears to be a major turning point in the lives of the three people with schizophrenia. Without the symptom relief provided by antipsychotic medications, CRO involvement would likely have been substantially reduced or nonexistent for Nick, Sue, and Mary.

If medications can play such a fundamental role in helping people overcome mental health problems, one may ask why it is even worth examining the social aspects of recovery. While medications certainly help tremendously, they do not help people overcome all mental health problems. Even if drugs worked perfectly and prevented people from experiencing any sort of symptom distress, the social aspects of recovery would remain essential. Drugs will never provide a sense of love, belonging, or friendship. These feelings are fundamental to mental health and they can only be obtained through social interaction. Medications help to make productive social interaction possible, but drugs in isolation cannot create productive social interactions.

Furthermore, medications can work wonders but they do not work perfectly. Mary, Nick, and Sue still face formidable limitations as a result of their mental health problems. CROs provide a unique social environment that can accommodate these limitations, thereby allowing people to pursue rewarding lives.

Consistent with the consumer recovery model, the self-directed nature of CRO participation and organizational operation appears to facilitate recovery. The P.S. Club's continued operation required leadership effort on the part of several members. As described in Chap. 6, this leadership involvement helped to promote resource exchange, skill development, favorable self-appraisals, and identity transformation. These changes, in turn, promote recovery, as described in Chaps. 2 and 3. The self-directed nature of social and recreational involvement provides members with opportunities to find others who have faced similar challenges and cultivate mutually supportive friendships. These friendships can promote recovery by serving as helping resources, where people can obtain emotional support in times of need and learn effective coping strategies others have successfully used.

It is important to note that some progress toward recovery attributable to CRO participation depends on continued CRO participation, whereas other progress toward recovery transcends CRO participation and carries over into other contexts. Specifically, enhancements in the quality and meaningfulness of life that rely on increased activity and resource exchanges from role development at a CRO will deteriorate if the CRO roles are lost. However, the skill development and identity transformations that grow out of involvement in challenging new roles can continue to contribute to recovery after CRO participation ends.

For people whose lives are dominated by dependency roles, these more permanent changes are needed to develop a sense of empowerment and responsibility for self-care. The identity transformation from dependent and helpless to independent and competent is difficult to achieve, but it is critical in the development of a meaningful life focused on self-actualization. However, some people may be content with a life full of satisfying recreation. For example, Kevin was not focused on personal growth or personal responsibility for self-care, but he was content with his recreation-focused life. The recovery model does not provide clear guidance on whether or how Kevin could make progress toward recovery. Based on the principle of self-determination, he was living a life he selected that he found satisfying. However, Kevin's livelihood depended on government assistance and he was not interested in taking action to become more independent. It is difficult to know whether attempts to change his lifestyle would be helpful, and what attempts at intervention would need to look like in order to be effective.

Summary Implications for Practice

A thorough understanding of how people benefit from CROs can help guide the development of effective CROs. The development of effective strategic plans to enhance CRO effectiveness requires understanding how people benefit so that appropriate change processes can be targeted by the strategic plans. Understanding the outcomes associated with well-run CROs and the processes by which people benefit can help CRO leaders and allies explain the benefits to potential CRO participants, and write more compelling funding applications to support CROs. The following sections discuss in more detail some of the key insights gleaned from this book that can help CRO stakeholders develop more effective CROs.

Developing Challenging New Roles

One of the key insights gained from the life-history narratives is that skill development and identity transformation will only occur if people take on new roles that challenge their current skill set and self-conceptualization. Thus, settings that want to promote skill development and identity transformation need to find ways to engage people in challenging new roles. Our understanding of how to do this is largely underdeveloped and future research is needed. However, existing research and the life-history narratives themselves provide some insight into this issue.

At times, people simply need to be provided the opportunity to take on a challenging new role. For example, Sue was extremely ambitious and jumped at the chance to take on challenging roles such as CRO leader, full-time graduate student, and full-time employee. Readiness is an important individual characteristic to consider when encouraging people to engage in a challenging role. Sue's involvement in a CRO leadership role helped prepare her for her university studies, which in turn prepared her for her full time job. Each role was appropriately challenging, but risked being a set-up for failure accompanied by overwhelming stress without the personal growth had occurred in previous roles. It is important to ensure role opportunities are challenging without being overwhelming. For example, Nick was able to pursue his role as Director of the P.S. Club because he was able to back off and rest when he felt overwhelmed.

Sometimes role engagement may not be feasible. For example, Kevin was ready to engage in recreational activities but he expressed no interest in a leadership role at the P.S. Club. Despite encouragement from several members, Kevin always identified as a member but not a leader. Although it is difficult to know if Kevin could have been gradually engaged in leadership activities, others have responded well to gradually increasing leadership involvement. For example, Carl began his P.S. Club attendance by simply making friends with others. Gradually over time he began taking on leadership roles such as member of the Board of Directors, peer counseling coordinator, shift manager, and then President of the Board of Directors. Over time, his ownership of the club increased, as did his identity as a leader.

Readiness for Challenging New Roles

When trying to engage people in new roles, it is important to consider the conditions under which someone can be successful in a new role. For example, Laura was ready to engage in recreational activities and make friends, but only in a nonjudgmental environment where she would not be criticized. The P.S. Club provided such an environment and she grew attached quickly. Creating environments that accommodate the needs of members while avoiding conditions that caused past engagement failures is critical to successfully engaging individuals in new roles. Despite her severe mental health problems, Mary was able to successfully perform her duties as shift manager and Treasurer of the Board of Directors when she was feeling well. The only reason she was able to continue her leadership involvement at the P.S. Club is because it accommodated her need to be absent frequently.

Recreation and Social Support

Regardless of whether people take on new challenges, involvement in CROs can provide important benefits to participants. CRO involvement replaced time spent alone in front of the TV for several P.S. Club informants including Joe, Mary, Carl, Kevin, and Laura. Such engagement helped to provide members with enough roles and relationships to fill up their time and energy. Just as everyone needs active engagement in roles, people need rest and down time from role involvement. The self-directed nature of CRO participation helped people control their extent of role involvement.

Although recreational involvement was not a challenging role for many members, it nevertheless served as a rewarding activity. CROs can fill a niche in the community by providing people with mental health problems recreational activities. The lack of accommodating social settings can make it hard for many people with mental health problems to find a place outside the home where they are welcome and comfortable socializing. When developing settings, it is important to be responsive to the interests and needs of the target population so that they will want to engage. CROs are well suited to be responsive because they are operated by the target population.

The recreational activities CROs choose to organize help to provide stress relief and serve as a medium for developing friendships. It is important not to underestimate the power of exchanging jokes, compliments, recognition, and appreciation in promoting mental health. People with mental health problems are frequently socially isolated and struggle to maintain relationships. Having a familiar and reliable social outlet substantially improved the quality of life for several members including Carl, Mary, Kevin, Laura, and Joe.

Conflict

As evidenced by Joe's narrative, the gains in quality of life from having friends and a reliable social outlet are lost as soon as the friendships and social outlet are lost. Joe stopped participating in the P.S. Club because of unresolved conflicts with fellow P.S. Club members. Settings must have effective conflict resolution procedures in order to minimize the interpersonal strain caused by conflict. One strategy settings can use to minimize the negative consequences of conflict is a code of conduct, as discussed in more detail in Chap. 8.

Promoting the Development of Leadership and Friendship Roles

Results from the quantitative analyses presented in Chaps. 7 and 8 make it clear that CROs should work to encourage the development of both empowering leadership roles and socially supportive friendship roles. CROs can use several strategies to promote empowering leadership roles, such as emphasizing the use of participatory decision making processes and encouraging volunteer efforts. To encourage the development of socially supportive friendship roles, CROs can organize a variety of activities that spark the interest of their members and make a point to recognize member accomplishments and milestones. Chapter 8 provides a detailed discussion of these and other strategies CROs can use to promote the development of friendship and leadership roles.

It is important to note that friendship and leadership engagement strategies often complement one another. For example, CROs can encourage leadership involvement by getting many different members involved in organizing recreational activities. Having many leaders planning and organizing recreational activities can, in turn, promote socially supportive friendship roles, as new members engage in the new recreational activities and begin to make friends.

Organizational Size

Results from Chap. 7 suggest that larger CROs exclude more people from leadership roles. However, the larger organizational size does not inhibit the average members' recovery. In fact, larger CROs may be more successful because they have a larger number of leaders who are capable of organizing a broader variety of organizational activities. The idea of preferring large CROs over small CROs is not consistent with previous research by Zimmerman et al. (1991), who identified the creation of underpopulated settings as a successful expansion strategy used by GROW. This discrepancy could be due to several factors. First, the Zimmerman study focused on expanding the number of groups and did not examine whether the underpopulated groups were as effective in promoting recovery. Second, GROW is substantially different from the CROs studied in this book because it provides a model for operating self-help groups but does not attempt to organize activities outside of group meetings the way the drop-in centers studied in this book did. An underpopulated self-help group that does not need to raise money may be substantially less problematic than an underpopulated CRO that depends on grant funding for survival. It may be that creating new underpopulated CROs in underserved areas is a good expansion strategy, whereas splitting large CROs to ensure all CROs are underpopulated is misguided. It is important to note that an emphasis on expanding the number of CROs without ensuring each CRO has adequate leadership can compromise the sustainability of the CROs (Salem, Reischl, & Randall, 2008).

Strengths and Weaknesses of the Methods

This book provides insights into how people benefit from CROs through a critical analysis of the literature and from four studies. Chapters 1 and 2 synthesize the literature on CROs and how people can benefit from CRO involvement. Chapter 3 presents the first study designed to provide insight into how people benefit from CROs. The study used focused questions to inform the development of a more comprehensive theoretical framework that could capture the change processes and outcomes described by CRO participants. Chapters 4, 5, and 6 present the method, results, and conclusions of an ethnographic study that used life-history narratives to provide an in-depth, contextualized understanding of how CRO involvement altered the developmental trajectories of several CRO participants. Chapter 7 presented the results of a quantitative study examining how organizational size influences role and relationship development. Chapter 8 presents a follow-up quantitative analysis examining how empowering leadership roles and socially supportive friendship roles contribute to recovery. Each chapter considers some specific strengths and limitations of the methods used in each study. This concluding chapter compares the strengths and weaknesses of the different research strategies, providing a more holistic understanding of how they fit together.

From a theory development perspective, the first study was the most useful. Analyzing the responses of 194 CRO participants to focused questions about how they benefit from CRO participation provided a relatively comprehensive list of the relevant processes and outcomes, as understood by CRO participants. This list helped to identify gaps in the preliminary conceptual framework based solely on a critical review of the literature. A key limitation of this approach is that it did not provide a richly contextualized understanding of change processes. Instead, it generated many ideas that required organization first through categorization and then through integration into the role framework.

The strengths of the second study filled in for weaknesses of the first and vice versa. The ethnographic methods and life-history narratives provide a richly contextualized insider's perspective on how people benefit from CRO participation. The life-history narratives also help to strengthen the voice of marginalized populations by conveying an insider's perspective in a compelling manner. This contextual knowledge proved essential in understanding how the theorized change processes can unfold over time in different life situations. The small sample size limits the generalizability of the findings. However, the use of thick description helps to alleviate problems transferring findings to other settings. Readers can use the rich contextual information to make judgments about the transferability of findings from the study context to the conditions under which lessons learned may be applied (Lincoln & Guba, 1986).

A key advantage of the journalistic life-history narrative method is that it provides results that are accessible to a broader audience than just academic researchers. Dissemination of the narratives to students and practitioners can help to reduce the gap between science and practice. If the narratives are disseminated in mainstream news outlets, they can also raise awareness about issues under study, providing thoughtful, well-informed, in-depth coverage at a time when funding for such work in the field of journalism is dwindling (Isaacson, 2009). Such dissemination of an insiders' understanding of mental health problems and recovery can help strengthen the voice of a typically marginalized population. When attempting to disseminate to a nonacademic audience, visual materials supplementing the text are an important addition because they help to draw readers into the story and hold their attention (Wolf & Grotta, 1985). Strong photographs also help to tell the story by proving relevant contextual information and illustrating points made in the text.

The recovery narratives can also serve as inspiring stories for people who are struggling with similar mental health problems. The successes described in the narratives can provide guidance on recovery by sharing examples of how others have managed to overcome mental health problems. As a recovery tool, journalistic narratives have several advantages over other intervention strategies used to promote healthy behavior change (Hinyard & Kreuter, 2007; Kreuter et al., 2007). The narratives can provide healthy behavioral models that readers can easily relate to, reducing message resistance and improving self-efficacy to undertake similar behavior changes (Bandura, 1997; Knowles & Linn, 2004).

A key limitation of the life-history method is that it is only as accurate as the writer's understanding of the life history. I attempted to provide an accurate portrayal of the insiders' perspective through participant observation, but I am unable to fully understand the experience because I do not have severe mental health problems. My own subjective perspective and biases also influenced the narratives.

In fact, the entire ethnographic study can be seen as a product of my own subjective experience and perspective. The literature review and role framework represents the knowledge and perspective that I had at the beginning of the study. The data from interviews and participant observation are based on questions I asked and from what I observed people doing. Thus, the life-history narratives reflect what I learned about informants from my interactions with them. My analysis of narratives explores how my perspective relates to what I learned in the field, thereby enriching my understanding of how people benefit from CROs.

The quantitative studies have the advantage of being somewhat more systematically objective. Everyone answered the same questions using the same scale and the results of the analysis are based on an impartial statistical calculation. However, in quantitative studies researchers retain control over what questions are asked and how answers are analyzed. Thus, the framing of the investigation is far more tightly controlled by the researcher and the influence of the informants' perspective and ideas is minimized. Whereas the quantitative research allowed me to test existing ideas with planned statistical analyses, the qualitative research allowed me to generate new ideas by talking to people in an open-ended format.

A key limitation of the quantitative studies is their dependence on cross-sectional associations. Although I am interested in testing causal relations between the components of the role framework, I have yet to do so. Results from the analysis presented in Chaps. 7 and 8 are consistent with causal hypotheses, but provide no grounds for causal inference. Longitudinal studies that use random assignment are needed for causal inference, as discussed more fully in the next section.

Future Research Directions

The role framework provides a promising theoretical explanation of how people benefit from CRO participation and make progress toward recovery. The framework can help guide researchers into productive areas of inquiry, sharpening focus on insightful questions, appropriate analyses, and contextualized conclusions that help move our understanding of CROs forward. In particular, the role framework can inform the design of rigorous studies that test the effectiveness of CROs. The role framework can guide the selection of contextually appropriate outcome measures, along with relevant individual and setting characteristics that may influence outcomes. Further, the role framework specifies mediating interpersonal processes that are critical to outcome attainment and need to be measured in outcome evaluations.

Previously presented research indicates the role framework can coherently organize and describe the change processes and outcomes described by CRO participants. Quantitative studies examining parts of the role framework provide preliminary evidence of this feasibility as a causal model. Before embracing the role framework as an accurate description of how people benefit from CROs, its predictions need to be tested using rigorous quantitative methods. However, before testing the accuracy of the role framework's predictions, measures of the various role framework constructs need to be developed. The development of strong quantitative measures for role framework constructs is a major undertaking because of the abstract nature of the constructs. The development of quantitative measures requires construct specificity than is not provided by the role framework.

To begin, the idea that person–environment interaction (component 1) leads to role and relationship development (component 2) is intentionally vague so that it can describe a broad variety of persons interacting in numerous environments, which may lead to any number of roles and relationships. The personal, environmental, and role characteristics of interest must be specified before a prediction can be tested. Inevitably, roles will only develop under certain conditions. Future qualitative research needs to develop hypotheses about the relevant personal and environmental characteristics that lead to the development of certain types of roles. Future quantitative research needs to test the predictions.

Based on existing literature reviewed in Chap. 2 and the research presented in this book, I hypothesize that the following environmental characteristics of CROs influence role and relationship development:

- Organizational size (Chap. 7)
- Accepting or judgmental atmosphere (Chap. 6)
- Sense of community (Chavis & Wandersman, 1990)
- Internal conflict (Chap. 6)
- Empowering environment (Maton & Salem, 1995)
- Sharing of leadership responsibilities (Wituk, Shepherd, Warren and Meissen 2002)
- Number of planned social activities (Kaufmann, Ward-Colasante, and Farmer, 1993).

I hypothesize that the following individual characteristics influence role and relationship development within CROs. Chapter 2 discusses more fully the rationale and research supporting these hypotheses.

- Experiential knowledge of severe mental health problems (Borkman, 1999)
- Demographic characteristics including age, education, gender, and race/ethnicity

- Similarity between self and group
- Amount of social support outside the CRO

Specific roles must also be identified, defined, and measured. I hypothesize that empowering leadership roles and socially supportive friendship roles are two theoretically relevant roles in the CRO context. Chapter 8 provides a more complete discussion of these roles and the existing measurement limitations that need to be addressed in future research.

Substantial measurement development work is also needed to adequately assess the consequences of role and relationship development. Specifically, the resource exchange, skill development, and identity transformation that can result from involvement in friendship and leadership roles must be specified before measures can be identified or developed. Relevant resource exchanges in friendship roles are thought to include positive reflected appraisals such as compliments, laughter, and expressions of gratitude. People may also receive helpful information, emotional support, and tangible support in friendship roles. Within volunteer leadership roles, positive reflected appraisals may be the most important resource. In paid leadership roles, money is an important resource acquired by role inhabitants. With regard to skill development, friendship roles can enhance social skills whereas leadership roles can improve leadership skills. Fortunately, measures of both social skills (e.g., Lowe & Cautela, 1978) and leadership skills (e.g., Talbott & Hallows, 2008) exist in the literature. Similarly, several measures of self-esteem already exist (e.g., Rosenberg, 1965), thus making changes in self-appraisal relatively easy to measure. Identity transformation may be more difficult to capture with precision, but several strategies have been described in the literature (Callero, 1992; Siebert & Siebert, 2005; Stryker & Serpe, 1994). Once a general identity measurement strategy is selected, a specific measure needs to be developed. Identity transformations related to friendship role involvement would capture the extent to which individuals view themselves as friendly and sociable. The measurement of identity transformations related to leadership involvement is more debatable, but would likely involve capturing self-perceptions as someone whose ideas are worth sharing, who can make decisions with confidence, who has a strong vision for the future, and who wants to provide guidance to groups they are involved with.

Once strong measures for each of the role framework components are identified or developed, studies that rigorously test role framework predictions need to be designed and executed. However, randomized trials are difficult to execute effectively in CROs because the development of roles and relationships is highly dependent upon self-selection. The lack of control over role and relationship development at a CRO makes the use of random assignment difficult.

One strategy that may make random assignment more feasible is to use an intensive engagement intervention that can help ensure that someone will in fact develop roles and relationships at a CRO. Researchers could then randomly assign the intensive engagement intervention, thereby helping to reduce noncompliance among research participants assigned to the intervention condition. A simple referral is frequently too weak of an engagement intervention because people often do not comply with the recommendation. However, previous research has found the use of a sponsor outreach intervention to be an effective strategy for increasing the likelihood that referral will lead to attendance (Powell, Hill, Warner, Yeaton, & Silk, 2000; Sisson & Mallams, 1981). Supplementing in-person and phone contacts from group members with mailings and emails may also be helpful. Targeting person and environment characteristics that more likely interact in a manner that leads to role development can also help to improve rates of engagement in friendship and leadership roles within a randomized trial.

Researchers who randomly assign an intensive engagement intervention can examine whether it leads to role and relationship development, resource exchange, improved self-appraisal, skill development, and identity transformation. Mediation analyses can further examine the causal path from role development to resource exchange, self-appraisal, skill development, and identity transformation. Randomized trials that employ intensive engagement techniques also aid the development of effective outreach tactics. Research that provides insight into the engagement process is of great practical value because the most prominent needs of CROs and other self-help initiatives frequently center on member recruitment and engagement (Meissen, Gleason, & Embree, 1991).

Numerous other research strategies are equally promising. For example, longitudinal observational field studies can study the trajectories of different people who encounter CROs. Findings can provide insight into patterns of role and relationship development. Analyses can also help to identify the individual characteristics that make role development more or less likely. If enough CROs are included in these studies, analyses will be able to examine how environmental characteristics and person–environment interactions influence participation, outcomes, and sustainability. Such studies can aid the development of guidelines for ideal environmental characteristics that promote participation, group sustainability, and individual benefit.

Qualitative research also has the potential to make important contributions to our understanding of CROs. For example, in-depth interviews and focus groups can help to identify strategies for improving organizational operations and provide important insight into the creation of effective outreach materials. Interviews with CRO leaders and professionals who support CROs can help build understanding of how professionals can best interact with and support CROs. Given the lack of theoretical guidance in approaching these topics, they are ripe for development through qualitative techniques.

In all CRO studies, consumers who operate CROs need to be involved in the research process (Nelson, Ochocka, Griffin, & Lord, 1998). Only through close collaboration will research efforts succeed in developing and testing practical hypotheses that will help CROs become more successful. In the co-creation of research projects, it is important to reach consensus on several issues including the values guiding the partnership, the sharing of power and responsibility, the research focus, and how the knowledge will be used (Nelson, Janzen, Ochocka, & Trainor, 2010).

Closing Remarks

CROs are a low-cost strategy for promoting the well-being of mental health consumers (Holter & Mowbray, 2005; Segal, Silverman & Temkin 2010; Teague, Johnsen, Rogers and Schell 2005). The influence of CROs is likely to continue expanding in the foreseeable future, leading to dramatic changes in the mental health system. Most professional mental health services have consumer equivalents. Consumer case managers, counselors, and peer support specialists are becoming increasingly popular (Salzer, 2010; Solomon & Draine, 1995, 1996). The CROs studied in this book are similar to professionally run psychosocial clubhouses (Mowbray, Woodward, Holter, MacFarlane, & Bybee, 2009). Even psychiatric hospitalization could be replaced by consumer-run crisis residential services, which have been shown to be equally effective (Greenfield, Stoneking, Humphreys, Sundby, & Bond, 2008). The use of consumers as providers of mental health services is a radical departure from the traditional mental health system. Although CROs appear to be viable and effective, their penetration across communities is limited. Future work needs to develop effective dissemination models that can help to ensure the implementation of high-quality CROs. Although research can provide important guidance, it is important to remember that CRO implementation will always remain an art that science can only help to refine.

The role framework provides a compelling framework for understanding how people engage in and benefit from involvement in CROs and other community settings. It posits that the roles we develop determine the resources we receive, the skills we develop, the identity we adopt, and the self-appraisals we make. The roles we develop describe not only the behaviors we expect of ourselves, but also the behavioral responses we expect from those with whom we interact. Characteristics of the person and the environment interact to determine whether roles develop and what behavioral expectations make up these roles.

This relatively simple framework for understanding complex human behavior has some important implications. If we want to empower people to act independently and take responsibility for self-care, we must provide people with opportunities to voluntarily develop mutually supportive roles, in which they exchange resources with others as equals. In such egalitarian roles, people must give in order to receive. If the exchanges are not equal and role involvement is voluntary, individuals unsatisfied with what they are receiving will leave, seeking out more rewarding role relationships. In such an environment, people learn that they must find ways to help others in order to receive the resources they desire (whether the desired resources are emotional support, esteem, information, tangible services, goods, or money). CROs provide such an environment, where people help each other to get what they want.

The traditional mental health system provides an environment full of status differentials and dependency roles. People that want help have to prove they are incompetent, and thus worthy of receiving help without being helpful. In the long run however, people do not typically receive as much in dependency roles as they would in a helper role. Instead, they receive barely enough to survive, especially if they depend on the government.

The traditional mental health system capitalizes on the human desire to help those who are helpless. This desire is healthy in moderation, as nobody is healthy all the time and people do need help during recovery. At the same time, people must be given opportunities to help themselves by helping others; otherwise people risk becoming trapped in dependency roles. CROs stand as one opportunity where people with mental health problems can find egalitarian, mutually supportive roles.

It is striking how common the activities in a CRO are throughout the rest of a typical community. People interact through work and recreation activities. In these social interactions, healthy collaborative relationships form, such as that of friend or colleague. "Normal" people participate in these relationships every day. If "abnormal" people only experience the relationships at a CRO, and they seem to become mentally healthier as a result of these interactions, then it seems more emphasis on mutually supportive interactions will help people become "normal." If the paths to recovery and community integration is embodied in the development of mutually supportive roles, then perhaps we should focus on making sure people find this path earlier in life and avoid learning helplessness as a means of survival. The role framework suggests that as a society, we need to encourage voluntary involvement in mutually supportive relationships and discourage the development of dependency roles.

Appendix A

Organizational Health Questionnaire

Self-Help Network

Center for Community Support and Research
Wichita State University

CRO Member Survey
Name of Organization _____
Date _____

We're very excited to visit this place today. We want to hear what you have to say about your experiences here. Your individual answers are anonymous. Only the average response of the group will be shared with others. This information will not be used to make any funding decisions. There are no right or wrong answers to these questions as they are based on your opinion. If you have any questions while completing this, please feel free to ask at any time. We'll be glad to help!

First, Here Are Some Background Questions...

1. Sometimes mood can affect how you answer questions. Please circle the word that best describes how you feel today?
   Terrible-------Unhappy-------OK-------Happy-------Great
2. How long have you been coming here?
   – For a few weeks
   – For a couple of months
   – For more than six months (but less than a year)
   – For more than a year. How many years? _____
3. How often do you come here? Please check one box.
   – Every day
   – Several times a week
   – About once a week
   – A couple times per month
   – A few times per year
4. How hard is it for you to get here? Please check one box.
   – Very hard
   – Hard
   – Easy
   – Very easy
5. Are you female or male? Please check one: __ Male __ Female
6. Check one category that best describes your marital status right now.
   – Single (never married)
   – Married (or Domestic Partner)
   – Living with Boyfriend or Girlfriend
   – Separated
   – Widowed
   – Divorced
7. Please check all that apply
   – White/Caucasian
   – Black/African American
   – Asian or Pacific Islander
   – American Indian or Alaskan Native
   – Spanish or Hispanic
   – Other, please specify _____
8. What year were you born? _____
9. Please check all the forms of education you have completed.
   – Less than High School
   – Graduated from High School
   – G.E.D.
   – Technical training beyond high school
   – Some college
   – Graduated from college (ex. B.A.)
   – Graduate degree (ex. Masters)

10. What kind of place are you currently living in?
    - My own house/apartment – alone
    - My own house/apartment – with family or friends
    - Staying with friends (their place)
    - Staying with parents/relatives (their place)
    - Rooming or boarding house
    - Group home or adult foster care
    - No current residence (living in a shelter or on the streets)
    - Other (please specify) _____

Next, we have some questions about your experiences at this place.

How much do you agree with the following statements…

1.	I feel like I belong to the community here.	Not at All	A Little	A Lot
2.	I socialize with people from here at other places.	Not at All	A Little	A Lot
3.	The friendships I have with people here mean a lot to me.	Not at All	A Little	A Lot
4.	If something was being planned here, I'd join in.	Not at All	A Little	A Lot
5.	If I needed advice about something, I could go to someone here.	Not at All	A Little	A Lot
6.	I agree with most people here about what is important in life.	Not at All	A Little	A Lot
7.	I believe people here would help me in an emergency.	Not at All	A Little	A Lot
8.	I feel loyal to the people here.	Not at All	A Little	A Lot
9.	I borrow things and exchange favors with people here.	Not at All	A Little	A Lot
10.	I plan to keep involved with people from here for a number of years.	Not at All	A Little	A Lot
11.	I think of myself as similar to others here.	Not at All	A Little	A Lot
12.	I have people from here over to my place to visit.	Not at All	A Little	A Lot
13.	I regularly talk with other people here.	Not at All	A Little	A Lot

People participate in different ways at places like this. Here is a list of things that might be true about what you have done here. Please circle Yes or No for each question. Many people answer No to all the questions so do not feel bad about never doing the activities on this list.

1.	Have you voted in an election for Board members?	Yes	No
2.	Have you served on the Board of Directors here?	Yes	No
3.	Have you helped set up any meetings here?	Yes	No
4.	Have you been responsible for preparing meals or bringing refreshments here?	Yes	No
5.	Are you a volunteer on a regular basis here?	Yes	No
6.	Have you been a paid staff member here?	Yes	No
7.	Have you helped lead a discussion or support group here?	Yes	No
8.	Have you taken part in deciding what activities will be held here?	Yes	No
9.	Have you taken part in deciding whether to add a new program or service here?	Yes	No
10.	Have you taken part in deciding whether to hire someone?	Yes	No
11.	Have you taken part in deciding what rules people need to follow here?	Yes	No
12.	Have you taken part in deciding what to do if someone breaks the rules here?	Yes	No
13.	Have you suggested to the Board or director what you think might be changed or improved here?	Yes	No
14.	Have you taken part in writing the yearly grant here?	Yes	No
15.	Have you taken part in writing the quarterly reports here?	Yes	No
16.	Have you helped with cleaning or building maintenance here?	Yes	No
17.	Have you helped organize a fun activity or party here?	Yes	No
18.	Have you taught a class here?	Yes	No
19.	Have you designed or helped collect survey information (e.g., satisfaction survey, KU survey)?	Yes	No
20.	Have you attended an external meeting or conference for this organization?	Yes	No
21.	Have you made a presentation at an external meeting or conference for this organization?	Yes	No

Appendix A

For each of the following statements, please indicate whether you strongly agree, agree, neither agree nor disagree (i.e., neutral), disagree, or strongly disagree. Please compare your current situation to your life before you became involved in this organization.

	Since I have become involved here…	Strongly agree	Agree	Neutral	Disagree	Strongly disagree
1.	I deal more effectively with daily problems	SA	A	N	D	SD
2.	I feel better about myself	SA	A	N	D	SD
3.	I am better able to control my life	SA	A	N	D	SD
4.	I am better able to deal with a crisis	SA	A	N	D	SD
5.	I am getting along better with my family	SA	A	N	D	SD
6.	I do better in social situations	SA	A	N	D	SD
7.	I do better in school or work (if applicable)	SA	A	N	D	SD
8.	I do better with my leisure time (that is I get more out of leisure time)	SA	A	N	D	SD
9.	My housing situation has improved	SA	A	N	D	SD
10.	My symptoms are not bothering me as much	SA	A	N	D	SD
11.	I have become more independent	SA	A	N	D	SD
12.	I have become more effective in getting what I need	SA	A	N	D	SD
13.	I can deal better with people and situations that used to be a problem for me	SA	A	N	D	SD
14.	I use crisis mental health services less	SA	A	N	D	SD
15.	I use non-crisis mental health services less	SA	A	N	D	SD
16.	I have become more ambitious	SA	A	N	D	SD
17.	I have become more competent	SA	A	N	D	SD
18.	I have become more confident	SA	A	N	D	SD

Please indicate how much you agree or disagree with each statement about this organization

	Thinking about the qualities of this organization…	Strongly agree	Agree	Neutral	Disagree	Strongly disagree
1.	This place promotes learning, striving and growth	SA	A	N	D	SD
2.	This place has a hopeful environment that promotes positive expectations	SA	A	N	D	SD
3.	This place is inspiring and encouraging	SA	A	N	D	SD
4.	This organization provides opportunities for meaningful participation and contribution	SA	A	N	D	SD
5.	This place helps people feel valued and respected	SA	A	N	D	SD
6.	This place helps people feel connected to others in positive ways	SA	A	N	D	SD
7.	This place is safe	SA	A	N	D	SD
8.	There are creative and interesting things going on here	SA	A	N	D	SD
9.	This organization asks for member feedback	SA	A	N	D	SD
10.	This organization makes changes based on member input and satisfaction	SA	A	N	D	SD
11.	This organization provides leadership opportunities	SA	A	N	D	SD

12. What personal changes have occurred as a result of your involvement here?

13. What experiences did you have here that enabled personal change?

Appendix A

The following questions are about mutual support, intimacy and sharing at your organization. Please indicate how true each of the following statements are.

	Thinking about the qualities of this organization…	Always true	Mostly true	Sometimes true	False
1.	The people who come here are proud of this place	AT	MT	ST	F
2.	This is a place where you can get help if you have a problem	AT	MT	ST	F
3.	Everybody here pitches in to help make this a good organization	AT	MT	ST	F
4.	People receive recognition and praise here when they have accomplished something	AT	MT	ST	F
5.	People can learn about housing, social security and other useful information here	AT	MT	ST	F
6.	A lot of day to day problems are solved here	AT	MT	ST	F
7.	People who come here are learning to depend on themselves more	AT	MT	ST	F
8.	This is a place where you can find out what is happening around town (meetings, events, etc.)	AT	MT	ST	F
9.	This is a place where you can talk about your hopes and dreams	AT	MT	ST	F
10.	People at this place feel close to each other	AT	MT	ST	F
11.	This is a place to share feelings without being put down	AT	MT	ST	F
12.	This is a good place to share your ideas with people	AT	MT	ST	F
13.	This is a good place to be yourself	AT	MT	ST	F

14. At this place, how many people can you talk to about personal things? _____ people
15. Outside of this place, how many people can you talk to about personal things? _____ people
16. If a friend were in need of similar help, would you recommend this organization to him/her?
    – No, definitely not
    – No, I don't think so
    – Yes, I think so
    – Yes, definitely
17. In an overall, general sense, how satisfied are you with this organization?
    – Very Satisfied
    – Mostly Satisfied
    – Indifferent or mildly dissatisfied
    – Quite dissatisfied

Here are some questions about conflict and the rules at this organization. Please circle the word that best describes your opinion.

1. Are there rules at this organization? Circle YES or NO
2. How familiar are you with the rules here?

    Not Familiar-----------Somewhat Familiar------------Very Familiar

3. How often were these rules violated or ignored in the past three months?

    Not Once-------Very Seldom--------About Half-------Quite Often-------All the Time
    The Time

4. How clear are the consequences to breaking the rules?

    Not Clear----------Somewhat Clear----------Very Clear

5. How consistently are these rules enforced?

    Not Enforced------Loosely Enforced------Usually Enforced------Always Enforced

6. How satisfied are you with the rules at this organization?

    Very Satisfied------Satisfied------Indifferent------Dissatisfied------Very Dissatisfied

7. During the past 3 months how often did disagreements or arguments occur?

    Not Once------About Once------About Once------Several Times------Several Times
    A Month   A Week   A Week   A Day

8. How often do people stay away from this organization because of conflict?

    Not At All--------A Little--------Some--------Quite A Bit--------All the Time

9. In general, when disagreements or arguments occurred, how often were they handled in each of the following ways during the past 3 months:

		Almost never	Seldom	About half the time	Often	Very Often
a.	By ignoring or avoiding the issues	AN	S	HT	O	VO
b.	By bringing the issues out in the open and working them out among the people involved	AN	S	HT	O	VO
c.	By having a paid staff member resolve the issues between the people involved	AN	S	HT	O	VO
d.	By enforcing the code of conduct	AN	S	HT	O	VO

Thanks for sharing your valuable thoughts and opinions! Your participation in this project will help others to create and improve organizations like this one.

Appendix B

Organizational Activity Survey

Self-Help Network
Center for Community Support and Research
Wichita State University

CRO Activity Survey
Name of Organization _____
Date _____

We're very excited to visit this place today. We are interested in learning more about consumer run organizations, so we're coming to the experts-the people who come here. We want to hear what you have to say about your experiences here. There are no right or wrong answers to these questions; we just want know about all the different things your organization is doing. If you have any questions while completing this, please feel free to ask at any time. We'll be glad to help!

Appendix B

1. In the following [table?] please list the positions or titles of all *paid* employees at your CRO and the number of hours that individual works every week.

	Employee position	Hours worked per week	Briefly describe the roles and responsibilities of this employee below	Circle Gender
1		____ hours		Male / Female
2		____ hours		Male / Female
3		____ hours		Male / Female
4		____ hours		Male / Female
5		____ hours		Male / Female
6		____ hours		Male / Female

2. The following table asks about member involvement in your organization's reporting and management activities. Please estimate the number of people who help with each activity described below.

Reporting or management activity	Circle the approximate number of members who are involved in this activity
Completing SRS quarterly reports	[1–2] [3–4] [5–6] [7–8] [9–10] [11+]
Completing the yearly SRS grant	[1–2] [3–4] [5–6] [7–8] [9–10] [11+]
Financial reporting such as taxes	[1–2] [3–4] [5–6] [7–8] [9–10] [11+]
Making and changing the budget	[1–2] [3–4] [5–6] [7–8] [9–10] [11+]
Making decisions about who gets hired	[1–2] [3–4] [5–6] [7–8] [9–10] [11+]

3.

Circle the approximate number of members who are involved in any activity related to reporting and management	[1–3] [4–6] [7–9] [10–14] [15–20] [21+]

4.

Circle the approximate number of members who are involved in planning and organizing all of the different activities your CRO provides for its members	[1–3] [4–6] [7–9] [10–14] [15–20] [21+]

5.

Circle the approximate number of paid staff and volunteers who are involved in a support role at your organization such as cleaning, preparing food, building maintenance and transportation assistance. This does not include work where people are planning or organizing an event	[1–5] [6–10] [11–20] [21–30] [31–50] [50+]

Here Are Some Questions About Your Board of Directors...

1. How many consumers are on your board of directors? _____ consumers
2. How many non-consumers are on your board of directors? _____ non-consumers
3. How many vacancies are on your board of directors? _____ positions
4. Do you have board officer positions that are vacant? Circle YES or NO
   If YES then which office positions are vacant?
   Circle PRESIDENT VICE PRESIDENT TREASURER SECRETARY
5. How often does your board meet? _____ times a year
6. Is a financial statement ever distributed to the board when you meet? Circle YES or NO
   If YES how often is the financial statement distributed to the board? _____ times a year
   Please attach a copy of your most recent financial statement.
7. Do you vote on all major expenses? Circle YES or NO
8. Are minutes taken at your board meetings? Circle YES or NO
   If YES are minutes distributed to board members after the meeting? Circle YES or NO
9. Is an agenda provided to board members at the beginning of a board meeting? Circle YES or NO
10. Do you have an annual meeting to elect board members? Circle YES or NO
11. Does your board evaluate your executive director? Circle YES or NO
12. Have you ever had problems getting a quorum? Circle YES or NO
    If YES, about how many times a year does this occur? _____ times a year
13. Do you have a code of conduct or other behavior policies in place? Circle YES or NO
    If YES, what percentage of the time are these policies enforced? _____ % of the time

Finally, Here Are Some Questions About Member Satisfaction and Attendance...

1. Does your CRO have a suggestion box where members can leave comments or complaints? Circle YES or NO
2. Does your CRO administer a satisfaction questionnaire? Circle YES or NO
   If YES, how often do you administer the questionnaire? _____ times a year
3. Does your CRO conduct focus groups to assess member satisfaction? Circle YES or NO
   If YES, how often do you conduct focus groups? _____ times a year
4. Are you currently working to increase membership or attendance? Circle YES or No

If YES, what are you doing to increase membership or attendance?
_____
_____
_____

5. Are you currently working to increase public awareness of your CRO? Circle YES or NO
   If YES, what are you doing to increase public awareness?
   _____
   _____
   _____

6. Are there any other projects or activities that your organization is involved in that you would like us to know about? Circle YES or NO
   If YES please describe them below:
   _____
   _____
   _____

Thanks for sharing your valuable thoughts and opinions! Your participation in this project will help create and improve organizations like this one.

Appendix C

Minimally Structured Interview Questions

Introduce the Study Before Each Interview

Describe the purpose of the interview
About how long the interview will take
Recording info
Read through the informed consent
Answer any questions participant may have

Interview Segment 1: Personal Background

Educational history
    What would you say were the best things about school?
    What would you say were the worst things about school?
    Describe to me a typical school day growing up.
Religious background
    What role does religion play in your life?
        Describe your experiences with church.
Residential history
    Could you list all the different towns you have lived in.
        How long did you live in (old residence)
        How is (old residence) different from (current residence)?
        Why did you decide to leave?
Aspects of upbringing
    Could you describe your living conditions growing up.
    Tell me about what a typical weekend growing up was like.
    What events in your life have had the biggest influence on your development?

Employment history
    Could you list all the different jobs you have had.
    Tell me about your job as a (job name).
        What would you say were the best things about that job?
        What would you say were the worst things about that job?

Mental illness history.
    Do you consider yourself to have a mental illness?
    What does having a mental illness mean to you?
    What do you think having a mental illness means to other people?
    Tell me about your mental illness
        When did you realize something was wrong?
        What did you do?
        What symptoms do you have?
    How has it changed your life?
        How does it make life more difficult?
        Could you give me an example of how having a mental illness caused you problems?
        What is the most frustrating aspect of having mental illness?
How do others respond when they find out you have a mental illness?
Is there anything you want to teach others about what it is like to have a mental illness?
How do you cope with your mental illness?
How has your experience with the illness changed over the years?
Tell me about the mental health services you use.
    Which ones do you use?
    What are they like?
    What do you like about the services?
    How do you benefit from the services?
    What would you change about the services?

Interview Segment 2: Community Participation Experiences

How did you end up in (town)?
What would you say are the best things about living in (town)?
What would you say are the worst things about living in (town)?
Tell me about a typical day living in (town).
Tell me about a good day.
    What makes a day good in your mind?
    Do other good day stories come to mind?
Tell me about a bad day.
    What makes a day bad in your mind?
    Do other bad day stories come to mind?
What is it like to live in (town)?

Appendix C

What are people like around here?
Tell me about your neighbors.
     What do you talk about?
What do you do around here?
   Do you ever go shopping around here?
   Do you work?
   Do you go to church?
   Are you involved in any community groups?
   Do you do any volunteer work?
   What do you do for fun around here?
What do you enjoy doing most?
Who do you enjoy spending time with? Why?
What activities are most involved in these days?
   Are there any activities outside of your involvement in the P.S. Club that you have taken on since joining?
   What challenges do you face in your daily life? (e.g. finances, transportation, access to health care)
Now think back to (year), just before you joined the P.S. Club.
   How was your typical day different then from what it is now?
      Were there any everyday problems that you have since resolved?
      Have any new problems arisen in that time frame?
      What did you have less time for once you started going to the P.S. Club?
      What activities were you involved in then that you are not involved in now?

CRO Participation Experiences

How did you first get started with the P.S. Club?
Why do you come to the P.S. Club?
   How does this place benefit you?
   How would you describe the P.S. Club?
Tell me about a typical visit here.
   What do you do around here?
   Tell me about a good experience you had here.
   Tell me about a bad experience you had here.
How would you describe the atmosphere here?
   What do you do to influence the atmosphere here?
Do you feel like coming here has changed you? How?
What experiences have you had here that enabled personal change?
   Do you feel like you have met people who are like you, that understand you? Are these people different from regular everyday people? How so?
How have the relationships that you have formed here benefited you?
Have you ever helped someone at the P.S. Club? How?
Have you ever been helped by someone at the P.S. Club? How?

A bringer of new things; and vile it were
For some three suns to store and hoard myself,
And this gray spirit yearning in desire
To follow knowledge like a sinking star,
Beyond the utmost bound of human thought.

This is my son, mine own Telemachus,
To whom I leave the scepter and the isle—
Well-loved of me, discerning to fulfill
This labour, by slow prudence to make mild
A rugged people, and through soft degrees
Subdue them to the useful and the good.
Most blameless is he, centered in the sphere
Of common duties, decent not to fail
In offices of tenderness, and pay
Meet adoration to my household gods,

When I am gone. He works his work, I mine.
There lies the port; the vessel puffs her sail:
There gloom the dark broad seas. My mariners,
Souls that have toiled, and wrought, and thought with me—
That ever with a frolic welcome took
The thunder and the sunshine, and opposed
Free hearts, free foreheads—you and I are old;
Old age had yet his honour and his toil;
Death closes all: but something ere the end,
Some work of noble note, may yet be done,
Not unbecoming men that strove with Gods.
The lights begin to twinkle from the rocks:
The long day wanes: the slow moon climbs: the deep
Moans round with many voices. Come, my friends,
'Tis not too late to seek a newer world.
Push off, and sitting well in order smite
The sounding furrows; for my purpose holds
To sail beyond the sunset, and the baths
Of all the western stars, until I die.
It may be that the gulfs will wash us down:
It may be we shall touch the Happy Isles,
And see the great Achilles, whom we knew.
Though much is taken, much abides; and though
We are not now that strength which in the old days
Moved earth and heaven; that which we are, we are,
One equal-temper of heroic hearts,
Made weak by time and fate, but strong in will
To strive, to seek, to find, and not to yield.

References

Anthony, W. A. (1993). Recovery from mental illness: the guiding vision of the mental health service system in the 1990s. *Psychosocial Rehabilitation Journal, 16*, 11–23.

Bandura, A. (1997). *Self-efficacy: The exercise of control.* New York: Freeman.

Barker, R. G. (1968). *Ecological psychology.* Stanford, CA: Stanford University Press.

Bellack, A. S. (2006). Scientific and consumer models of recovery in schizophrenia: concordance, contrasts, and implications. *Schizophrenia Bulletin, 32*, 432–442.

Berkman, L. F., Glass, T., Brissette, I., & Seeman, T. (2000). From social integration to health: Durkheim in the new millennium. *Social Science & Medicine, 51*, 843–857.

Berkow, P. (2001). *English composition faculty guide for Annenberg/CPB telecourse.* New York: McGraw-Hill.

Blau, P. M. (1970). A formal theory of differentiation in organizations. *American Sociological Review, 35*, 210–218.

Blumer, H. (1969). *Symbolic interactionism: Perspective and method.* Englewood Cliffs, NJ: Prentice-Hall.

Borkman, T. J. (1999). *Understanding self-help/mutual aid: Experiential learning in the commons.* New Brunswick, NJ: Rutgers University Press.

Bright, J. I., Baker, K. D., & Neimeyer, R. A. (1999). Professional and paraprofessional group treatments for depression: a comparison of cognitive-behavioral and mutual support interventions. *Journal of Consulting and Clinical Psychology, 67*(4), 491–501. doi:10.1037/0022-006x.67.4.491.

Brown, L. D. (2004). *Goal achievement in mutual support organizations operated by persons with psychiatric disability. Masters Project.* Wichita, KS: Wichita State University.

Brown, L. D. (2009a). How people can benefit from mental health consumer-run organizations. *American Journal of Community Psychology, 43*, 177–188.

Brown, L. D. (2009b). Making it sane: using life history narratives to explore theory in a mental health consumer-run organization. *Qualitative Health Research, 19*, 243–257.

Brown, L. D., Collins, V. L., Shepherd, M. D., Wituk, S. A., & Meissen, G. (2004). Photovoice and consumer-run mutual support organizations. *International Journal of Self-Help and Self-Care, 2*, 339–344.

Brown, L. D., Shepherd, M. D., Merkle, E. C., Wituk, S. A., & Meissen, G. (2008). Understanding how participation in a consumer-run organization relates to recovery. *American Journal of Community Psychology, 42*, 167–178.

Brown, L. D., Shepherd, M. D., Wituk, S. A., & Meissen, G. (2007a). Goal achievement and the accountability of consumer-run organizations. *The Journal of Behavioral Health Services and Research, 34*, 73–82.

Brown, L. D., Shepherd, M. D., Wituk, S. A., & Meissen, G. (2007b). How settings change people: applying behavior setting theory to consumer-run organizations. *Journal of Community Psychology, 35*, 399–416.

Brown, L. D., Shepherd, M. D., Wituk, S. A., & Meissen, G. (2008). Introduction to the special issue on mental health self-help. *American Journal of Community Psychology, 42*, 105–109.
Brown, L. D., & Wituk, S. A. (Eds.). (2010). *Mental health self-help: Consumer and family initiatives*. New York: Springer.
Bruner, J. (1987). Life as narrative. *Social Research, 54*, 11–32.
Bryson, J. M. (1995). *Strategic planning for profit and nonprofit organizations: A guide to strengthening and sustaining organizational achievement*. San Francisco: Jossey-Bass.
Burke, P. J. (1991). Identity processes and social stress. *American Sociological Review, 56*(6), 836–849.
Burke, P. J. (2003). Introduction. In P. J. Burke, T. J. Owens, R. Serpe, & P. A. Thoits (Eds.), *Advances in identity theory and research* (pp. 1–7). New York: Kluwer/Plenum.
Burke, P. J., Owens, T. J., Serpe, R., & Thoits, P. A. (Eds.). (2003). *Advances in identity theory and research*. New York: Kluwer/Plenum.
Burkholder, G., & Harlow, L. (2003). An illustration of a longitudinal cross-lagged design for larger structural equation models. *Structural Equation Modeling, 10*, 465–486.
Burti, L., Amaddeo, F., Ambrosi, M., Bonetto, C., Cristofalo, D., Ruggeri, M., et al. (2005). Does additional care provided by a consumer self-help group improve psychiatric outcome? A study in an Italian community-based psychiatric service. *Community Mental Health Journal, 41*(6), 705–720. doi:10.1007/s10597-005-6428-1.
Callero, P. L. (1992). The meaning of self-in-role: a modified measure of role identity. *Social Forces, 71*, 485–501.
Camisón-Zornoza, C., Lapiedra-Alcamí, R., Segarra-Ciprés, M., & Boronat-Navarro, M. (2004). A meta-analysis of innovation and organizational size. *Organization Studies, 25*(3), 331–361. doi:10.1177/0170840604040039.
Carling, P. J. (1995). *Return to community: Building support systems for people with psychiatric disabilities*. New York: Guilford.
Center for Community Support & Research. (2003). An analysis of consumer-run organization quarterly reports. http://www.kansascro.com/includes/downloads/article_feedback.pdf. Acessesed 10 March 2009
Center for Community Support & Research. (2004). *Network analysis of consumer-run organizations*. Wichita, KS: Wichita State University Center for Community Support & Research.
Chamberlin, J. (1977). *On our own*. Lawrence, MA: National Empowerment Center.
Chamberlin, J. (1990). The ex-patients' movement: where we've been and where we're going. *Journal of Mind and Behavior, 11*, 323–336.
Chamberlin, J., Rogers, E. S., & Ellison, M. L. (1996). Self-help programs: a description of their characteristics and their members. *Psychiatric Rehabilitation Journal, 19*(3), 33–42.
Chavis, D. M., & Wandersman, A. (1990). Sense of community in the urban environment: a catalyst for participation and community development. *American Journal of Community Psychology, 18*, 55–81.
Chien, W.-T., Chan, S., Morrissey, J., & Thompson, D. (2005). Effectiveness of a mutual support group for families of patients with schizophrenia. *Journal of Advanced Nursing, 51*(6), 595–608. doi:10.1111/j.1365-2648.2005.03545.x.
Chien, W.-T., Chan, S. W. C., & Thompson, D. R. (2006). Effects of a mutual support group for families of Chinese people with schizophrenia: 18-month follow-up. *The British Journal of Psychiatry, 189*(1), 41–49. doi:10.1192/bjp.bp. 105.008375.
Chien, W.-T., Norman, I., & Thompson, D. R. (2006). Perceived benefits and difficulties experienced in a mutual support group for family carers of people with schizophrenia. *Qualitative Health Research, 16*(7), 962–981.
Chien, W.-T., Thompson, D. R., & Norman, I. (2008). Evaluation of a peer-led mutual support group for Chinese families of people with schizophrenia. *American Journal of Community Psychology, 42*(1–2), 122–134. doi:10.1007/s10464-008-9178-8.
Chiu, M. Y. L., Ho, W. W. N., Lo, W. T. L., & Yiu, M. G. C. (2010). Operationalization of the SAMHSA model of recovery: a quality of life perspective. *Quality of Life Research: An*

International Journal of Quality of Life Aspects of Treatment, Care & Rehabilitation, 19(1), 1–13. doi:10.1007/s11136-009-9555-2.

Clark, C. C., & Krupa, T. (2002). Reflections on empowerment in community mental health: giving shape to an elusive idea. *Psychiatric Rehabilitation Journal, 25*, 341–349.

Clay, S. (2005). About us: what we have in common. In S. Clay (Ed.), *On our own, together: peer programs for people with mental illness*. Nashville, TN: Vanderbilt University Press.

Clay, S., Schell, B., Corrigan, P. W., & Ralph, R. O. (2005). *On our own, together: peer programs for people with mental illness*. Nashville, TN: Vanderbilt University Press.

Coates, D., & Winston, T. (1983). Counteracting the deviance of depression: peer support groups for victims. *Journal of Social Issues, 39*, 169–194.

Cobb, S. (1976). Social support as moderator of life stress. *Psychosomatic Medicine, 38*, 300–314.

Coffman, D. L., & MacCallum, R. C. (2005). Using parcels to convert path analysis models into latent variable models. *Multivariate Behavioral Research, 40*, 235–259.

Cohen, S., Gottlieb, B. H., & Underwood, L. G. (2000). Social relationships and health. In S. Cohen, L. G. Underwood, & B. H. Gottlieb (Eds.), *Social support measurement and intervention: a guide for health and social scientists* (pp. 3–28). Oxford, England: Oxford University Press.

Cohen, S., & Wills, T. A. (1985). Stress, social support and the buffering hypothesis. *Psychological Bulletin, 95*, 310–357.

Connolly, P. M., & York, P. J. (2002). Evaluating capacity-building efforts for nonprofit organizations. *OD Practitioner, 34*, 33–39.

Constantino, V., & Nelson, G. (1995). Changing relationships between self-help groups and mental health professionals: shifting ideology and power. *Canadian Journal of Community Mental Health, 14*(2), 55–70.

Cooley, C. H. (1902). *Human nature and the social order*. New York: Charles Scribner.

Corrigan, P. W., Slopen, N., Gracia, G., Phelan, S., Keogh, C. B., & Keck, L. (2005). Some recovery processes in mutual-help groups for persons with mental illness; II: qualitative analysis of participant interviews. *Community Mental Health Journal, 41*(6), 721–735. doi:10.1007/s10597-005-6429-0.

COSP. (2000). Consumer Operated Service Program (COSP) multi-site baseline protocol 2.3 Retrieved August 1, 2006, from http://www.cstprogram.org/consumer%20op/Multi-Site%20Activities/Common%20Protocol/BaselineProtocol.pdf

Cowan, C. P., & Cowan, P. A. (1986). A preventive intervention for couples becoming parents. In C. Z. Boukydis (Ed.), *Research on support for parents and infants in the postnatal period*. New York: Ablex.

Deegan, P. E. (1988). Recovery: the lived experience of rehabilitation. *Psychosocial Rehabilitation Journal, 11*(4), 11–19.

Dees, J. G., & Economy, P. G. (2001). Social entrepreneurship. In J. G. Dees & P. G. Economy (Eds.), *Enterprising nonprofits* (pp. 1–19). New York: Wiley.

DeGarmo, D. S. (2010). A time varying evaluation of identity theory and father involvement for full custody, shared custody, and no custody divorced fathers. *Fathering, 8*(2), 181–202. doi:10.3149/fth.1802.181.

Dewar, R., & Hage, J. (1978). Size, technology, complexity, and structural differentiation: toward a theoretical synthesis. *Administrative Science Quarterly, 23*, 111–136.

Dickerson, F. B. (1998). Strategies that foster empowerment. *Cognitive and Behavioral Practice, 5*, 255–275.

Dollard, J. (1935). *Criteria for the life history*. New Haven, CT: Yale University Press.

Dunkel-Schetter, C. (1984). Social support and cancer: findings based on patient interviews and their implications. *Journal of Social Issues, 40*, 77–98.

Erikson, E. (1950). *Childhood and society*. New York: Norton.

Estroff, S. E. (1985). *Making it crazy: An ethnography of psychiatric clients in an American community*. Berkley, CA: University of California Press.

Festinger, L. (1954). A theory of social comparison processes. *Human Relations, 7*, 117–140.
Fischer, C. S. (1982). *To dwell among friends: Personal networks in town and city*. Chicago: University of Chicago Press.
Fisher, D., & Spiro, L. (2010). Finding and using our voice: how consumer/survivor advocacy is transforming mental health care. In L. D. Brown & S. Wituk (Eds.), *Mental health self-help: Consumer and family initiatives* (pp. 213–233). Springer Science+Business Media: New York, NY.
Flynn, R. J., & Lemay, R. A. (Eds.). (1999). *A quarter-century of normalization and social role valorization: Evolution and impact*. Ottawa, ON: University of Ottawa Press.
Foa, U. G., & Foa, E. B. (1974). *Societal structures of the mind*. Springfield, IL: Thomas.
Friedlander, E. J., & Lee, J. (2004). *Feature writing for newspapers and magazines: The pursuit of excellence* (5th ed.). Boston: Pearson Education.
Gidron, B., & Chesler, M. (1994). Universal and particular attributes of self-help: a framework for international and intranational analysis. In F. Lavoie, T. Borkman, & B. Gidron (Eds.), *Self-help and mutual aid groups: International and multicultural perspectives*. New York: Haworth.
Goldberg, R. W., Rollins, A. L., & Lehman, A. F. (2003). Social network correlates among people with psychiatric disabilities. *Psychiatric Rehabilitation Journal, 26*, 393–402.
Goldstrom, I. D., Campbell, J., Rogers, J. A., Lambert, D. B., Blacklow, B., Henderson, M. J., et al. (2006). National estimates for mental health mutual support groups, self-help organizations, and consumer-operated services. *Administration and Policy in Mental Health and Mental Health Services Research, 33*, 92–103.
Gourieroux, C., Holly, A., & Monfort, A. (1982). Likelihood ratio test, wald test, and kuhn-tucker test in linear models with inequality constraints on the regression parameters. *Econometrica, 50*, 63–80.
Greenfield, T. K., Stoneking, B. C., Humphreys, K., Sundby, E., & Bond, J. (2008). A randomized trial of a mental health consumer-managed alternative to civil commitment for acute psychiatric crisis. *American Journal of Community Psychology, 42*(1–2), 135–144. doi:10.1007/s10464-008-9180-1.
Hammer, M. (1981). Social supports, social networks, and schizophrenia. *Schizophrenia Bulletin, 7*, 45–57.
Hardiman, E. R. (2007). Referral to consumer-run programs by mental health providers: a national survey. *Community Mental Health Journal, 43*(3), 197–210. doi:10.1007/s10597-006-9079-y.
Hardiman, E. R., & Segal, S. P. (2003). Community membership and social networks in mental health self-help agencies. *Psychiatric Rehabilitation Journal, 27*, 25–33.
Hardy, C., Phillips, N., & Lawrence, T. (2003). Resources, knowledge and influence: the organizational effects of interorganizational collaboration. *Journal of Management Studies, 40*, 289–315.
Harper, G. W., Lardon, C., Rappaport, J., Bangi, A. K., Contreras, R., & Pedraza, A. (2004). Community narratives: the use of narrative ethnography in participatory community research. In L. A. Jason, C. B. Keys, Y. Suarez-Balcazar, R. R. Taylor, & M. I. Davis (Eds.), *Participatory community research: Theories and methods in action* (pp. 199–217). Washington, DC: American Psychological Association.
Helgeson, V. S., & Gottlieb, B. H. (2000). Support groups. In S. Cohen, L. G. Underwood, & B. H. Gottlieb (Eds.), *Social support measurement and intervention: A guide for health and social scientists* (pp. 221–245). Oxford, England: Oxford University Press.
Helgeson, V. S., & Mickelson, K. D. (1995). Motives for social comparison. *Personality and Social Psychology Bulletin, 21*, 1200–1209.
Heller, K. (1989). The return to community. *American Journal of Community Psychology, 17*, 1–15.
Hewitt, J. P. (2003). *Self and society: A symbolic interactionist social psychology*. Boston, MA: Allyn & Bacon.
Hinyard, L. J., & Kreuter, M. W. (2007). Using narrative communication as a tool for health behavior change: a conceptual, theoretical, and empirical overview. *Health Education and Behavior, 34*, 777–792.

Holter, M. C., & Mowbray, C. T. (2005). Consumer-run drop-in centers: program operations and costs. *Psychiatric Rehabilitation Journal, 28*, 323–331.

Holter, M. C., Mowbray, C. T., Bellamy, C. D., MacFarlane, P., & Dukarski, J. (2004). Critical ingredients of consumer run services: results of a national survey. *Community Mental Health Journal, 40*(1), 47–63.

Hox, J. J., & Maas, C. J. M. (2001). The accuracy of multilevel structural equation modeling with pseudobalanced groups and small samples. *Structural Equation Modeling, 8*, 157–174.

Humphreys, K., Mavis, B., & Stofflemayr, B. (1991). Factors predicting attendance at self-help groups after substance abuse treatment: preliminary findings. *Journal of Consulting and Clinical Psychology, 59*, 591–593.

Humphreys, K., & Woods, M. D. (1994). Researching mutual-help group participation in a segregated society. In T. J. Powell (Ed.), *Understanding the self-help organization: Frameworks and findings*. Thousand Oaks, CA: Sage.

Iorio, S. H. (2004). Focused interviews. In S. H. Iorio (Ed.), *Qualitative research in journalism: Taking it to the streets* (pp. 109–125). Mahwah, NJ: Lawrence Erlbaum Associates Publishers.

Isaacson, W. (2009). How to save your newspaper. *Time, 16*, 30–33.

Israel, B. A., House, J. S., Schurman, S. J., Heaney, C. A., & Mero, R. P. (1989). The relation of personal resources, participation, influence, interpersonal relationships, and coping strategies to occupational stress, job strains and health: a multivariate analysis. *Work and Stress, 3*, 163–194.

James, W. (1950). *The principles of psychology, Vol. 2*. New York: Dover. original work published, 1890.

Janzen, R., Nelson, G., Trainor, J., & Ochocka, J. (2006). A longitudinal study of mental health consumer/survivor initiatives: Part 4–Benefits beyond the self? A quantitative and qualitative study of system-level activities and impacts. *Journal of Community Psychology, 34*, 285–303.

Johnsen, M., Teague, G. B., & Herr, E. M. (2005). Common ingredients as a fidelity measure for peer-run programs. In S. Clay, B. Schell, P. W. Corrigan, & R. O. Ralph (Eds.), *On our own, together: Peer programs for people with mental illness* (pp. 213–238). Nashville, TN: Vanderbilt University Press.

Kaplan, B. H. (1980). *Deviant behavior in defense of self*. New York: Academic.

Kasinsky, J. (1987). Cooptation. In S. Zinman, H. T. Harp, & S. Budd (Eds.), *Reaching across: Mental health clients helping each other* (pp. 177–181). Sacramento, CA: California Network of Mental Health Clients.

Kaufmann, C. L., Ward-Colasante, C., & Farmer, J. (1993). Development and evaluation of drop-in centers operated by mental health consumers. *Hospital and Community Psychiatry, 44*, 675–678.

Kendell, R. E. (1975). The concept of disease and its implications for psychiatry. *The British Journal of Psychiatry, 127*, 305–315.

Kimura, M., Mukaiyachi, I., & Ito, E. (2002). The House of Bethel and consumer-run businesses: an innovative approach to psychiatric rehabilitation. *Canadian Journal of Community Mental Health, 21*(2), 69–77.

Kiresuk, T. J., & Lund, S. H. (1978). Goal attainment scaling. In C. C. Attkisson, W. A. Hargreaves, M. J. Horowitz, & J. E. Sorensen (Eds.), *Evaluation of human service programs*. New York: Academic.

Kishton, J. M., & Widaman, K. F. (1994). Unidimensional versus domain representative parceling of questionnaire items: an empirical example. *Educational and Psychological Measurement, 54*, 757–765.

Knowles, E. S., & Linn, J. (Eds.). (2004). *Resistance and persuasion*. Mahwah, NJ: Lawrence Erlbaum Associates.

Kreuter, M. W., Green, M. C., Capella, J. N., Slater, M. D., Wise, M. E., Storey, D., et al. (2007). Narrative communication in cancer prevention and control: a framework to guide research and application. *Annals of Behavioral Medicine, 33*, 221–235.

LeCompte, M. D., & Schensul, J. J. (1999). *Analyzing and interpreting ethnographic data*. Walnut Creek, CA: AltaMira.
Lee, D. L. (1988). The support group training project. In B. H. Gottlieb (Ed.), *Marshaling social support: Formats, processes, and effects* (pp. 135–163). Beverly Hills, CA: Sage.
Lewin, K. (1948). *Resolving social conflicts*. New York: Harper and Brothers.
Lieberman, M. A. (1993). Self-help groups. In H. I. Kaplan & B. J. Sadock (Eds.), *Comprehensive group therapy*. Baltimore, MD: Williams & Wilkins.
Lincoln, Y. S., & Guba, E. G. (1986). But is it rigorous? Trustworthiness and authenticity in naturalistic evaluation. *Naturalistic Evaluation, 30*, 73–84.
Linton, R. (1936). *The study of man*. New York: D. Appleton-Century.
Lowe, M. R., & Cautela, J. R. (1978). A self-report measure of social skill. *Behavior Therapy, 9*, 535–544.
Lucksted, A., Stewart, B., & Forbes, C. (2008). Benefits and changes for family to family graduates. *American Journal of Community Psychology, 42*, 154–166.
Luke, D. A., Roberts, L., & Rappaport, J. (1993). Individual, group context, and individual-group fit predictors of self-help group attendance. *The Journal of Applied Behavioral Science, 29*, 216–238.
Luks, A. (1991). *The helping power of doing good: The health and spiritual benefits of helping others*. New York: Fawcett Columbine.
Magura, S., Laudet, A. B., Mahmood, D., Rosenblum, A., & Knight, E. (2002). Adherence to medication regimens and participation in dual-focus self-help groups. *Psychiatric Services, 53*(3), 310–316. doi:10.1176/appi.ps.53.3.310.
Mankowski, E. S., Humphreys, K., & Moos, R. H. (2001). Individual and contextual predictors of involvement in twelve-step self-help groups after substance abuse treatment. *American Journal of Community Psychology, 29*, 537–563.
Mankowski, E. S., & Rappaport, J. (2000). Narrative concepts and analysis in spiritually-based communities. *Journal of Community Psychology, 28*(5), 479–493. doi:10.1002/1520-6629(200009)28:5<479::aid-jcop2>3.0.co;2-0.
Maretzki, T. (1973). Preface. In L. Nader & T. Maretzki (Eds.), *Cultural illness and health*. Washington, DC: American Anthropological Association Publication 9.
Maton, K. I., & Salem, D. A. (1995). Organizational characteristics of empowering community settings: a multiple case study approach. *American Journal of Community Psychology, 23*, 631–656.
McAdams, D. P. (1985). *Power, intimacy, and the life story: Personological inquiries into identity*. Homewood, IL: Dorsey.
McAdams, D. P. (1993). *The stories we live by: Personal myths and the making of the self*. New York: William Morrow.
McCall, G. J., & Simmons, J. L. (1978). *Identities and interactions: An examination of human associations in everyday life*. New York: Free Press.
McLean, A. H. (2000). From ex-patient alternatives to consumer options: consequences of consumerism for psychiatric consumers and the ex-patient movement. *International Journal of Health Services, 30*(4), 821–847.
McMillan, D. W., & Chavis, D. M. (1986). Sense of community: a definition and theory. *Journal of Community Psychology, 14*(6–23).
McMillan, B., Florin, P., Stevenson, J., Kerman, B., & Mitchell, R. E. (1995). Empowerment praxis in community coalitions. *American Journal of Community Psychology, 23*, 699–727.
Mead, G. H. (1934). *Mind, self, and society*. Chicago, IL: University of Chicago Free Press.
Medvene, L. J. (1990). Family support organizations: the functions of similarity. In T. J. Powell (Ed.), *Working with self-help* (pp. 120–140). Silver Spring, MD: National Association of Social Work.
Medvene, L. J., Lin, K. M., Wu, A., Mendoza, R., Harris, N., & Miller, M. (1994). Mexican American and Anglo American parents of the mentally ill: attitudes and participation in family support groups. *Prevention in Human Services, 11*, 141–163.
Medvene, L. J., Volk, F. A., & Meissen, G. (1997). Communal orientation and burnout among self-help group leaders. *Journal of Applied Social Psychology, 27*, 262–278.

Meissen, G. J., Gleason, D. F., & Embree, M. G. (1991). An assessment of the needs of mutual-help groups. *American Journal of Community Psychology, 19*, 427–442.
Menard, S. (2002). *Longitudinal research* (2nd ed.). Thousand Oaks, CA: Sage.
MHSIP. (2000). MHSIP Consumer Survey, Version 1.1 Retrieved August 1, 2006, from http://www.mhsip.org/MHSIP_Adult_Survey.pdf
Milofsky, C. (1988). *Community organizations: Studies in resource mobilization and exchange.* New York: Oxford University Press.
Mohr, W. K. (2004). Surfacing the life phases of a mental health support group. *Qualitative Health Research, 14*, 61–77.
Moos, R. H. (1974). *Evaluating treatment environments: A social ecological approach.* New York: Wiley.
Moos, R. H., & Humphrey, B. (1974). *Group environment scale form.* Palo Alto, CA: Consulting psychologists.
Mowbray, C. T., Chamberlin, P., Jennings, M., & Reed, C. (1988). Consumer-run mental health services: Results from five demonstration projects. *Community Mental Health Journal, 24*, 151–156.
Mowbray, C. T., Greenfield, A., & Freddolino, P. P. (1992). An analysis of treatment services provided in group homes for adults labeled mentally ill. *The Journal of Nervous and Mental Disease, 180*, 551–559.
Mowbray, C. T., Robinson, E. A., & Holter, M. C. (2002). Consumer drop-in centers: operations, services, and consumer involvement. *Health and Social Work, 27*, 248–261.
Mowbray, C. T., & Tan, C. (1993). Consumer-operated drop-in centers: evaluation of operations and impact. *Journal of Mental Health Administration, 20*, 8–19.
Mowbray, C. T., Woodward, A. T., Holter, M. C., MacFarlane, P., & Bybee, D. (2009). Characteristics of users of consumer-run drop-in centers versus clubhouses. *Journal of Behavioral Health Services and Research, 36*(3), 361–371. doi:10.1007/s11414-008-9112-8.
Muthén, L. K., & Muthén, B. O. (2006). *Mplus (Version 4.2) [Computer software].* Los Angeles, CA: Muthén and Muthén.
Muthén, L. K., & Muthén, B. O. (2007). *Mplus (Version 51) [Computer software].* Los Angeles, CA: Muthén & Muthén.
Muthén, B. O., & Satorra, A. (1995). Complex sample data in structural equation modeling. In P. V. Marsden (Ed.), *Sociological Methodology* (pp. 267–316). American Sociological Association: Washington, DC.
Nelson, G., Janzen, R., Ochocka, J., & Trainor, J. (2010). Participatory action research and evaluation with mental health self-help initiatives: a theoretical framework. In L. D. Brown & S. A. Wituk (Eds.), *Mental health self-help: Consumer and family initiatives* (pp. 39–60). New York: Springer.
Nelson, G., Lord, J., & Ochocka, J. (2001). *Shifting the paradigm in community mental health: Towards empowerment and community.* Toronto, Canada: University of Toronto Press.
Nelson, G., Ochocka, J., Griffin, K., & Lord, J. (1998). 'Nothing about me, without me': Participatory action research with self-help/mutual aid organizations for psychiatric consumer/survivors. *American Journal of Community Psychology, 26*(6), 881–912. doi:10.1023/a:1022298129812.
Nelson, G., Ochocka, J., Janzen, R., & Trainor, J. (2006). A longitudinal study of mental health consumer/survivor initiatives: Part 2–A quantitative study of impacts of participation on new members. *Journal of Community Psychology, 34*, 261–272.
Nelson, G., Walsh-Bowers, R., & Hall, G. B. (1998). Housing for psychiatric survivors: values, policy, and research. *Administration and Policy in Mental Health, 25*, 55–62.
Noordsy, D., Torrey, W., Mueser, K., Mead, S., O'Keefe, C., & Fox, L. (2002). Recovery from severe mental illness: an interpersonal and functional outcome definition. *International Review of Psychiatry, 14*, 318–326.
Norcross, J. C. (2000). Here comes the self-help revolution in mental heath. *Psychotherapy: Theory, Research, Practice, Training, 37*(4), 370–377.
Perkins, D. V., Burns, T. F., Perry, J. C., & Nielsen, K. P. (1988). Behavior setting theory and community psychology: an analysis and critique. *Journal of Community Psychology, 16*, 355–372.

Peterson, N. A., & Zimmerman, M. A. (2004). Beyond the individual: toward a nomological network of organizational empowerment. *American Journal of Community Psychology, 34*, 129–145.
Piaget, J. (1952). *The origins of intelligence in children*. New York: International University Press.
Pistrang, N., Barker, C., & Humphreys, K. (2008). Mutual help groups for mental health problems: a review of effectiveness studies. *American Journal of Community Psychology, 42*(1–2), 110–121. doi:10.1007/s10464-008-9181-0.
Plummer, K. (1983). *Documents of Life*. London: Unwin Hyman.
Polkinghorne, D. E. (1988). *Narrative knowing and the human sciences*. Albany, NY: State University of New York Press.
Polkinghorne, D. E. (1995). Narrative configuration in qualitative analysis. *International Journal of Qualitative Studies in Education, 8*, 5–23.
Powell, T. J., Hill, E. M., Warner, L., Yeaton, W., & Silk, K. R. (2000). Encouraging people with mood disorders to attend a self-help group. *Journal of Applied Social Psychology, 30*, 2270–2288.
QSR. (2002). *NUD*IST 6 [Computer software]*. Doncaster, Australia: QSR International.
Rabinow, P., & Sullivan, W. M. (1979). *Interpretive social science: A reader*. Berkley, CA: University of California Press.
Rappaport, J. (1995). Empowerment meets narrative: listening to stories and creating settings. *American Journal of Community Psychology, 23*(5), 795–807. doi:10.1007/bf02506992.
Raudenbush, S. W., & Bryk, A. S. (2002). *Hierarchical linear models* (2nd ed.). Newbury Park, CA: Sage.
Recovery International. (2009). History of Recovery International. From http://www.recovery-inc.org/about/history.asp. Accessed 29 August 2009.
Riessman, F. (1965). The "helper" therapy principle. *Social Work, 10*, 27–32.
Riessman, F., & Carroll, D. (1995). *Redefining self-help*. San Francisco: Jossey-Bass.
Riley, A., & Burke, P. J. (1995). Identities and self verification in the small group. *Social Psychology Quarterly, 58*, 61–73.
Roberts, L. J., Salem, D., Rappaport, J., Toro, P. A., Luke, D. A., & Seidman, E. (1999). Giving and receiving help: interpersonal transactions in mutual-help meetings and psychosocial adjustment of members. *American Journal of Community Psychology, 27*(6), 841–868. doi:10.1023/a:1022214710054.
Rodgers, R., & Hunter, J. E. (1991). Impact of management by objectives on organizational productivity. *Journal of Applied Psychology, 76*, 322–336.
Rook, K. (1990). Stressful aspects of older adults' social relationships: current theory and research. In J. H. Crowther, S. E. Hobfoll, & D. L. Tennenbaum (Eds.), *Stress and coping in later-life families* (pp. 221–250). New York: Hemisphere.
Rook, K. (1992). Detrimental aspects of social relationships: taking stock of an emerging literature. In H. O. Viel & U. Baumann (Eds.), *The meaning and measurement of social support* (pp. 157–169). New York: Hemisphere.
Rosenberg, M. (1965). *Society and the adolescent self-image*. Princeton, NJ: Princeton University Press.
Rosenberg, P. P. (1984). Support groups: a special therapeutic entity. *Small Group Behavior, 15*, 173–186.
Sabin, J. E., & Daniels, N. (2003). Managed care: Strengthening the consumer voice in managed care: VII. The Georgia peer specialist program. *Psychiatric Services, 54*(4), 497–498.
Salem, D., Reischl, T., & Randall, K. (2008). The effect of professional partnership on the development of a mutual-help organization. *American Journal of Community Psychology, 42*(1), 179–191. doi:10.1007/s10464-008-9193-9.
Salzer, M. S. (1997). Consumer empowerment in mental health organizations: concept, benefits, and impediments. *Administration and Policy in Mental Health, 24*, 425–435.
Salzer, M. S. (2010). Certified peer specialists in the United States behavioral health system: an emerging workforce. In L. D. Brown & S. Wituk (Eds.), *Mental health self-help: Consumer and family initiatives* (pp. 169–191). Springer Science+Business Media: New York, NY US.

References

Salzer, M. S., & Shear, S. L. (2002). Identifying consumer-provider benefits in evaluations of consumer-delivered services. *Psychiatric Rehabilitation Journal, 25*(3), 281–288.

Sarbin, T. R. (1966). Role Theory. In B. J. Biddle & E. J. Thomas (Eds.), *Role theory: Concepts and research*. New York: Wiley.

Sarbin, T. R. (1986). The narrative as a root metaphor for psychology. In T. R. Sarbin (Ed.), *Narrative psychology: The storied nature of human conduct* (pp. 3–21). Westport, CT: Praeger Publishers/Greenwood Publishing Group.

Schank, R. C., & Abelson, R. P. (1995). Knowledge and memory: the real story. In R. S. Wyer Jr. (Ed.), *Knowledge and memory: The real story* (pp. 1–85). Hillsdale, NJ England: Lawrence Erlbaum Associates, Inc.

Schoggen, P. (1989). *Behavior settings: a revision and extension of Roger G. Barker's Ecological Psychology*. Stanford, CA: Stanford University Press.

Schulz, A. J., Israel, B. A., Zimmerman, M. A., & Checkoway, B. N. (1995). Empowerment as a multi-level construct: perceived control at the individual, organizational and community levels. *Health Education Research, 10*, 309–327.

Segal, S. P., & Silverman, C. J. (2002). Determinants of client outcomes in self-help agencies. *Psychiatric Services, 53*, 304–309.

Segal, S. P., Silverman, C. J., & Temkin, T. L. (1993). Empowerment and self-help agency practice for people with mental disabilities. *Social Work, 38*, 705–712.

Segal, S. P., Silverman, C. J., & Temkin, T. L. (1995). Measuring empowerment in client-run self-help agencies. *Community Mental Health Journal, 31*, 215–227.

Segal, S. P., Silverman, C., & Temkin, T. (1997). Program environments of self-help agencies for persons with mental disabilities. *Journal of Mental Health Administration, 24*, 456–464.

Segal, S. P., Silverman, C. J., & Temkin, T. L. (2010). Self-help and community mental health agency outcomes: a recovery- focused randomized controlled trial. *Psychiatric Services, 61*(9), 905–910. doi:10.1176/appi.ps.61.9.905.

Shepherd, G., Boardman, J., & Slade, M. (2008). *Making recovery a reality*. London: Sainsbury Centre for Mental Health.

Sherman, S. R., Frenkel, E. R., & Newman, E. S. (1986). Community participation of mentally ill adults in foster family care. *Journal of Community Psychology, 14*, 120–133.

Siebert, D. C., & Siebert, C. F. (2005). The caregiver role identity scale: a validation study. *Research on Social Work Practice, 15*, 204–212.

Sisson, R. W., & Mallams, J. H. (1981). The use of systematic encouragement and community access procedures to increase attendance at alcoholic anonymous and al-anon meetings. *The American Journal of Drug and Alcohol Abuse, 8*, 371–376.

Skovholt, T. M. (1974). The client as helper: a means to promote psychological growth. *The Counseling Psychologist, 4*, 58–64.

Smith, D. H. (2000). *Grassroots associations*. Thousand Oaks, CA: Sage.

Solomon, P. (2004). Peer support/peer provided services: underlying processes, benefits, and critical ingredients. *Psychiatric Rehabilitation Journal, 27*, 392–401.

Solomon, P., & Draine, J. (1995). The efficacy of a consumer case management team: 2-year outcomes of a randomized trial. *Journal of Mental Health Administration, 22*(2), 135–146. doi:10.1007/bf02518754.

Solomon, P., & Draine, J. (1996). Service delivery differences between consumer and nonconsumer case managers in mental health. *Research on Social Work Practice, 6*(2), 193–207. doi:10.1177/104973159600600204.

Sosulski, M. R., Buchanan, N. T., & Donnell, C. M. (2010). Life history and narrative analysis: feminist methodologies contextualizing black women's experiences with severe mental illness. *Journal of Sociology and Social Welfare, 37*(3), 29–57.

Spector-Mersel, G. (2010). Narrative research: time for a paradigm. *Narrative Inquiry, 20*(1), 204–224. doi:10.1075/ni.20.1.10spe.

Stets, J. E., & Cast, A. D. (2007). Resources and identity verification from an identity theory perspective. *Sociological Perspectives, 50*(4), 517–543. doi:10.1525/sop.2007.50.4.517.

Strauss, A., & Corbin, J. (1998). *Basics of qualitative research: techniques and procedures for developing grounded theory.* Thousand Oaks, CA: Sage.
Stryker, S. (1968). Identity salience and role performance. *Journal of Marriage and the Family, 4,* 558–564.
Stryker, S. (1980). *Symbolic interactionism: A social structural version.* Menlo Park, CA: Benjamin Cummings.
Stryker, S., & Burke, P. J. (2000). The past, present, and future of identity theory. *Social Psychology Quarterly, 63,* 284–297.
Stryker, S., & Serpe, R. T. (1994). Identity salience and psychological centrality: Equivalent, overlapping, or complementary concepts? *Social Psychology Quarterly, 57,* 16–35.
Suls, J., Martin, R., & Wheeler, L. (2002). Social comparison: why, with whom and with what effect? *Current Directions in Psychological Science, 11*(5), 159–163.
Swann, W. B. (1987). Identity negotiation: where two roads meet. *Journal of Personality and Social Psychology, 53,* 1038–1051.
Swann, W. B., Pelham, B. W., & Krull, D. S. (1989). Agreeable fancy or disagreeable truth? Reconciling self-enhancement and self-verification. *Journal of Personality and Social Psychology, 57,* 782–791.
Swarbrick, M. (2007). Consumer-operated self-help centers. *Psychiatric Rehabilitation Journal, 31,* 76–79.
Talbott, B. H., & Hallows, S. (2008). Leadership skills: developing a measure for college students. *Intuition, 4,* 12–18.
Taylor, S. E. (1983). Adjustment to threatening events: a theory of cognitive adaptation. *The American Psychologist, 38,* 1161–1173.
Teague, G. B., Ganju, V., Hornik, J. A., Johnson, J. R., & McKinney, J. (1997). The MHSIP mental health report card: a consumer-oriented approach to monitoring the quality of mental health plans. *Evaluation Review, 21,* 330–341.
Teague, G.B., Johnsen, M., Rogers, J.A., & Schell, B. (2005). Research on consumer-operated service programs: Effectiveness findings and policy implications of a large multi-site study. Retrieved March 10 2009, from http://www.power2u.org/cosp.html.
Thoits, P. A. (1983). Multiple identities and psychological well-being. *American Sociological Review, 49,* 174–187.
Thoits, P. A. (1985). Social support and psychological well-being: theoretical possibilities. In I. G. Sarason & B. R. Sarason (Eds.), *Social support: Theory, research, and applications* (pp. 51–72). Dordrecht, The Netherlands: Martinus Nijhoff Publishers.
Thoits, P. A. (1986). Multiple identities: examining gender and marital status differences in distress. *American Sociological Review, 51,* 259–272.
Thoits, P. A. (2010). Stress and health: major findings and policy implications. *Journal of Health and Social Behavior, 51*(1 Suppl), S41–S53. doi:10.1177/0022146510383499.
Thoits, P. A., & Virshup, L. K. (1997). Me's and we's: forms and functions of social identities. In R. D. Ashmore & L. Jussim (Eds.), *Self and identity* (pp. 106–133). New York: Oxford University Press.
Thornton, T., & Lucas, P. (2011). On the very idea of a recovery model for mental health. *Journal of Medical Ethics: Journal of the Insitute of Medical Ethics, 37*(1), 24–28. doi:10.1136/jme.2010.037234.
Toseland, R. W., & Rossiter, C. M. (1989). Group interventions to support family caregivers: a review and analysis. *Gerontologist, 29,* 438–448.
Trainor, J., Shepherd, M., Boydell, K. M., Leff, A., & Crawford, E. (1997). Beyond the service paradigm: the impact and implications of consumer/survivor initiatives. *Psychiatric Rehabilitation Journal, 21,* 132–140.
Ullman, J. B. (2001). Structural equation modeling. In B. G. Tabachnick & L. S. Fidell (Eds.), *Using multivariate statistics* (4th ed.). Boston: Allyn and Bacon.
Unger, D. G., & Wandersman, A. (1985). The importance of neighbors: the social, cognitive, and affective components of neighboring. *American Journal of Community Psychology, 13,* 139–169.

Van Tosh, L., & del Vecchio, P. (2000). *Consumer-operated self-help programs: A technical report.* Rockville, MD: U.S. Center for Menal Health Services.
Veterans Health Administration. (2004). *VA Mental Health Strategic Plan.* Washington, D.C.: Office of Mental Health Services.
Wandersman, L., Wandersman, A., & Kahn, S. (1980). Social support in the transition to parenthood. *Journal of Community Psychology, 8,* 332–342.
Wang, C. C., & Burris, M. (1997). Photovoice: concept, methodology, and use for participatory needs assessment. *Health Education & Behavior, 24,* 369–387.
Wang, C. C., & Redwood-Jones, Y. A. (2001). Photovoice ethics: perspectives from Flint photovoice. *Health Education & Behavior, 28,* 560–572.
Whyte, W. (1980). *The social life of small urban spaces.* New York: Project for Public Spaces, Inc.
Wicker, A. W. (1991). Behavior settings reconsidered: temporal stages, resources, internal dynamics, context. In D. Stokols & I. Altman (Eds.), *Handbook of environmental psychology* (pp. 613–653). Malabar, FL: Krieger Publishing Company.
Wicker, A. W., McGrath, J. E., & Armstrong, G. E. (1972). Organization size and behavior setting capacity as determinants of member participation. *Behavioral Science, 17,* 499–513.
Wills, T. A. (1981). Downward comparison principles in social psychology. *Psychological Bulletin, 90,* 245–271.
Wills, T. A. (1985). Supportive functions of interpersonal relationships. In S. Cohen & S. L. Syme (Eds.), *Social support and health* (pp. 61–82). New York: Academic.
Wituk, S. A., Shepherd, M. D., Warren, M., & Meissen, G. (2002). Factors contributing to the survival of self-help groups. *American Journal of Community Psychology, 30,* 349–366.
Wituk, S. A., Vu, C., Brown, L. D., & Meissen, G. (2008). Organizational capacity needs of consumer-run organizations. *Administration and Policy in Mental Health and Mental Health Services Research, 35,* 212–219.
Wolf, R., & Grotta, G. L. (1985). Images: a question of readership [Article]. *Newspaper Research Journal, 6*(2), 30–36.
Wong, Y. I., & Solomon, P. L. (2002). Community integration of persons with psychiatric disabilities in supportive independent housing: a conceptual model and methodological considerations. *Mental Health Services Research, 4*(1), 13–28.
Wothke, W. (2000). Longitudinal and multi-group modeling with missing data. In T. D. Little, K. U. Schnabel, & J. Baumert (Eds.), *Modeling longitudinal and multilevel data: Practical issues, applied approaches, and specific examples.* Mahwah, NJ: Lawrence Erlbaum Associates.
Wuthnow, R. (1994). *Sharing the journey: Support groups and America's new quest for community.* New York: Free Press.
Yanos, P. T., Primavera, L. H., & Knight, E. L. (2001). Consumer-run service participation, recovery of social functioning, and the mediating role of psychological factors. *Psychiatric Services, 52,* 493–500.
Zimmerman, M. A., & Rappaport, J. (1988). Citizen participation, perceived control, and psychological empowerment. *American Journal of Community Psychology, 16,* 725–750.
Zimmerman, M. A., Reischl, T. M., Seidman, E., Rappaport, J., Toro, P. A., & Salem, D. A. (1991). Expansion strategies of a mutual help organization. *American Journal of Community Psychology, 19,* 251–278.

Index

A
Anxiety, 28, 44, 63, 82, 120, 164

B
Behavior setting theory, 13–16, 20–22, 33, 138, 140, 143–145, 147–150

C
Certified peer specialist training programs, 6
Code of conduct, 162–163, 171
Community integration
 physical integration, 5, 16, 18–20
 psychological integration, 5, 16, 18–20
 social integration, 16, 18–20
Community relations, 12
Community treatment/rehabilitation paradigm, 4, 5
Conflict, 10, 11, 125, 132, 152, 162–163, 171, 175
Conflict resolution, 10, 44, 126, 163, 171
Consumer-delivered services, 4, 6
Consumer movement, 10
Consumer-operated self-help centers, 4
Consumer-operated services, 4, 6, 142
Consumer rights, 5, 22
Consumer-run drop-in centers, 4, 6
Consumer-run services, 4
Consumers as providers, 6, 9, 178
Consumer/survivor initiatives, 4
Consumer technical assistance centers, 6
Cooptation, 8, 11–12
Coping, 3, 7, 16, 18, 19, 23–26, 33, 39, 44–47, 52, 71, 129, 139, 140, 142, 152, 163, 164, 168
Crisis residential programs, 6

D
Deinstitutionalization, 3, 5, 65
Dependency roles, 1, 2, 19, 43–45, 80, 121–123, 134, 135, 153, 169, 178, 179
Depression, 5, 44, 63, 68, 72, 82, 95, 98, 99, 106, 109, 123, 129, 164
Documentary photography, 2, 13
Drop-in center, 2, 4, 6, 37, 54, 70, 95, 172

E
Emic, 59
Empowerment, 3, 5, 6, 11, 13, 16, 20, 22, 51, 115, 139, 147, 152–154, 157, 169
Empowerment/community integration paradigm, 4, 5, 17
Empowerment theory, 13, 15, 16, 20, 22–23, 29, 33, 151
Engagement, 2, 19, 22, 31, 42, 43, 49, 50, 53, 59, 84, 86, 100, 102, 125, 127, 128, 130, 132, 145, 147, 150, 154, 162, 169–172, 176–178
Ethnographic methods, 1, 2, 14, 50, 52, 173
Etic, 59, 60
Expectations, 1, 8, 13, 17, 25–28, 32, 33, 43–46, 52, 121, 123, 127, 133, 135, 144, 148, 151, 154, 163, 165, 178
Experiential knowledge, 13, 16, 17, 19, 20, 23–24, 29, 33, 46, 111, 152, 160, 161, 175

F
Focused questions methodology, 36–38
Friendship roles, 10, 14, 33, 42, 45, 46, 120–122, 124, 125, 129, 132–135, 146–148, 150–156, 158–160, 162–166, 171–173, 176, 177
Funding support, 2, 8, 11–12

G
Goal achievement, 7, 12
Goal tracking, 11, 12

H
Helper-therapy principle, 13, 16, 17, 22–23, 29, 33, 46
Help provider, 17, 19, 20, 27, 32, 40, 42, 146
Help seeker, 17, 19, 20, 27, 32
Hierarchy, 3, 8, 9, 21, 28, 29, 149
Hospitalization, 5–7, 24, 40, 70, 82, 112, 119, 130, 132, 134, 178

I
Identity theory, 13, 17, 26–29, 43, 57, 126
Identity transformation, 29, 30, 32–34, 38, 45, 46, 121, 123, 124, 126, 128, 129, 131, 134, 135, 139, 146, 152, 168, 169, 176, 177
Inter-organizational collaboration, 12
Interpersonal processes, 15–17, 22–26, 175

J
Journalistic methods, 2, 50, 52

L
Leadership, 7–10, 13, 14, 21–23, 29, 32, 37, 54, 56, 78, 79, 96, 101, 113, 115, 123, 125, 134, 137–140, 143, 145, 148, 149, 154, 160, 161, 165, 166, 168, 170–172, 175, 176
Leadership roles, 10, 13, 14, 16, 19, 21–23, 32, 33, 40, 42, 44–46, 76, 120, 121, 124–129, 132, 133, 135, 137–141, 143, 145–148, 150–156, 158–161, 163–166, 170–173, 176, 177
Leadership skills, 161, 176
Life history narratives, 2, 13, 14, 49–61, 63–117, 132–134, 168, 169, 173, 174

M
Medical/institutional paradigm, 4
Mental health policy, 15, 78
Mental health self-help, 3–6, 43
Minimally structured interviews, 49, 50, 57–59
Multilevel models, 2, 144, 165
Mutual support, 2, 3, 8, 37, 54, 70, 132

N
Narrative arc, 52, 60
Narrative construction, 14, 50, 52, 58–61
Narrative research, 50, 51

O
Organizational networks, 12
Organizational size, 8, 9, 14, 137, 138, 140, 141, 143–145, 147, 150, 172, 173, 175
Organizational structure, 2, 5, 8–10
Outcomes, 2, 3, 7, 15–20, 22, 26, 29, 34, 43, 132, 139, 146, 164, 165, 169, 172, 173, 175, 177
Overpopulation, 20, 33, 138, 143, 147, 148, 150

P
Paid employment, 7, 40, 41, 43
Participant observation, 14, 49, 50, 55–59, 174
Peer counseling, 45, 54, 76, 91, 97, 123, 163, 170
Peer-run organizations, 4
Peer-run programs, 4
Personal change, 12, 35–43, 47, 49, 50
Person-environment interaction, 30–31, 33, 41–42, 53, 119, 121, 123, 125–130, 132, 137, 138, 148, 159, 166, 175, 177
Photovoice, 55, 56, 100, 101
Plot, 59, 60

R
Randomized controlled trial (RCT), 5, 6, 176, 177
Recovery, 3, 5, 6, 11–18, 20, 22, 33, 34, 46, 47, 52, 59–61, 66, 72, 75, 78, 79, 86, 92, 93, 95, 96, 98, 112, 114, 116, 137, 139–147, 149–169, 172–174, 179
Recreational activities, 4, 40, 45, 65, 72, 89, 91, 100, 121, 125–128, 132, 147, 166, 170–172
Reflected appraisal, 44, 124, 129, 154, 176
Resource exchange, 41, 43, 45–47, 120, 122, 124, 125, 127, 128, 130, 133, 139, 146, 148–150, 152, 153, 168, 176–178
Role framework, 2, 13, 14, 33, 35–47, 49–61, 119, 132, 134, 137, 139, 145, 146, 148–150, 152, 153, 159, 167, 173–176, 178, 179

Roles, 1–5, 8–11, 13, 14, 16, 17, 19–23, 25–33, 35–47, 49–61, 76, 80, 89, 92, 93, 114, 116, 119–135, 137–179
Role skills, 32, 44, 121–124, 126, 127, 129, 131, 133

S

Schizophrenia, 63, 66, 68, 82, 86, 88, 93, 121, 168
Self-appraisal, 32, 41, 43, 44, 46, 47, 120, 122, 124, 126, 127, 129–131, 133, 139, 146, 148, 150, 152, 168, 176–178
Self-esteem, 16, 25, 29, 32, 33, 38, 39, 41, 44, 46, 76, 80, 83, 94, 95, 97, 98, 120–122, 124, 133, 135, 142, 160, 176
Self-help agencies, 4
Self-help groups, 2–5, 8, 13, 31, 163, 172
Self-help programs, 4
Sense of belonging, 16, 20, 24, 26, 45, 68, 134, 168
Sense of community, 3, 13, 15–17, 19–20, 22, 29, 31, 33, 175
Shared leadership, 8, 13, 161
Skill development, 30, 32, 33, 46, 57–60, 123, 133, 146, 152, 160, 168, 169, 176, 177
Social comparison theory, 13, 16, 17, 23–25, 33, 46
Social functioning, 7, 13, 22, 135, 139
Social isolation, 9, 24, 68, 164, 166
Social network, 16, 19, 25, 27, 31, 33, 38–40, 42, 46, 57, 58, 110, 128, 146, 154, 156, 158–159, 166
Social skills, 39, 44–46, 79, 91, 113, 122–124, 133, 134, 176
Social support (and socially supportive), 7, 13, 14, 16, 17, 23, 25–26, 29, 31, 33, 39–41, 43, 46, 65, 79, 111, 124, 130, 133–135, 146, 150–156, 158–166, 170–173, 176
Stigma, 5, 10, 23, 24, 28, 39, 68, 88, 123
Stress, 16, 19, 26, 39, 42, 43, 46, 71, 72, 85, 88, 89, 91, 116, 120, 122, 133, 152, 170, 171
Structural equation modeling, 3, 14, 155–158, 165
Sustainability, 13, 172, 177

T

Technical assistance, 6, 10, 12, 36, 54, 55, 57, 78, 115, 130, 159
Theory development, 35, 60, 173

U

Underpopulation, 21, 138, 143, 147, 148, 150

V

Visual storytelling, 50, 53
Volunteer opportunities, 160